Get Me Skinny!!

Tony Arreola

Disclaimer

Medical Disclaimer

This publication contains the ideas and opinions of its author. It is intended to provide helpful information on the subjects addressed in the publication. It is sold with the understanding that the author and the publisher are not engaged in rendering medical, health or any kind personal professional services in the book. The reader should consult his or her medical professional before adopting any of the suggestions in this book or drawing inferences from it. The author and publisher disclaim all responsibility for any liability, loss, or risk, personal or otherwise, which is incurred as a consequence, directly or indirectly, of the use and application of the contents of this book.

What if you had a secret?

A secret that could help everyone you've ever loved;

reach the body of their dreams.

Would you share it? I did ...

Claudia :)

I wanted to wish you much success on your fitness journey. I hope you find this book enjoyable and informative. I look forward to hearing of your fitness success.

Cheers to Health & Fitness!

Tony 2013 :)

Tony Arreola

CONTENTS

Preface   i

1 I Try, Try and Then Try Some More...   1

2 Who's This Skinny Guy Anyway?   6

3 Get Me Skinny!!   11

4 What in the World Is a Calorie?   16

5 Paging Dr. M   23

6 Oh, No!! What Is This?   33

7 You Will Fall ... Get Up!   40

8 The Little Voice   45

9 Drill Sergeant Dan   51

10 The MAD PLAN   59

11 Here We Go ... Day One ... (Again)   82

12 Saturday. No, Wait ... SATURDAAAYYYY!!   88

13 Good Ole Sunday Brunch   94

14 Move, Move, and Move Some More   97

15 Sweet, Sweet Success!!   105

    Appendix: Movement Program   117

    Exercise to Food Ratios   117

    Testimonials   118

    About the Author   120

    Stay Connected   121

Preface

Are you ready? Are you excited to finally possess the body of your dreams? I wrote this book for you-the yo-yo dieter, the gym quitter, the new mom, the bikini body dreamer, the New Year's Resolutioner, the diet pill taker, the person who has tried everything with little success. As a personal trainer, I realize there is a vast amount of weight loss information out there. It is hard to determine what one should do. But before we ask what we should do, we need to discover why we should do. We need to establish the foundation and the proper mental framework for a successful fitness program. Understanding fitness and the mind is the best way to achieve long term results. This book will teach the underlying motivators to help you discover the secret to sustained weight loss. It is designed to take the complicated and make it simple. To make weight loss a realistic goal, and have you enjoy the same success that hundreds of my clients have experienced.

I wrote this book for everyone that has been burned by the fitness industry. I have personally lost over fifty pounds and it saddens me to watch people who want to get in shape start with a faulty plan that has no chance of success. Although, they want to succeed, without the right approach or correct information, they have no chance. It is my hope that this book can educate and enlighten. People need to know that fitness is attainable and with an accurate approach, actually quite simple.

This book is different and this is why it will work. Not only is it based on sound and proven fitness macro principles, but it is presented in a quick, easy to read story designed to help present complex topics in a simple manner. You need to remember that fitness is meant to be fun; it's fitness, not a painful chore. Great health is a wonderful treasure that can be shared by everyone. With this new fitness knowledge, it can be.

First of all I would like to thank all of my clients. You are the reason I am able to do what I love. It is because of you that my life is completely fulfilled. Your success defines me and every single story is special to me. Every single one, I want you to know that it is because of your support and love that anything like this is even remotely possible. For that, I am eternally grateful.

I would also like to thank my family and friends. I have had memorable mentors, outstanding leaders, and treasured friendships that have shaped the better part of my life. You have always believed in me and my dreams. Thank you.

Finally and most importantly, I would like to thank my mother. She has been the steady rock in my life. As an immigrant, single mother of four, I am still amazed at her ability to endure, her resilience and most importantly, the love for her children. Thank you mom for believing in me, this is for you.

I Try, Try and Then Try Some More...

What happened? How did I let myself get like this? My life is spiraling out of control. I can remember those beautiful summer days when I was proud of my body. It seems like forever ago. Buying clothes is so depressing now. Nothing fits right and I want to cry every time I see that dreaded reflection in the mirror. I hide from old friends. I speed past mirrors. I can't even remember the last time I felt ... sexy. How did this happen? This wasn't supposed to be my life. I hate this feeling. Argh! I am so frustrated.

Aubrey prepared to leave spin class, loathing her body. She stopped dead in her tracks as she caught a glimpse of herself in the mirror. *I hate how I look. Is everyone staring at me? I bet they wonder what I'm doing here. Probably taking bets on how long before I quit.*

As Aubrey gathered her bag, she overheard a couple of skinny girls talking about their personal trainer.

"Can you believe I lost twenty-five pounds?" said one skinny girl.

"I know, and I lost thirty. And the craziest part is that it wasn't that hard," replied the other skinny girl.

"I'm grateful he was able to fit us into his schedule."

"I know. He's so busy."

As Aubrey left, she wondered who these skinny girls were talking about. *It must be some pompous, arrogant trainer that works at the gym*, she thought. Aubrey had awful experiences in the past with personal trainers and their tacky sales techniques. Being overweight, she felt like a target. She had no idea how overweight she was because she refused to climb on a scale. The mere thought of what the scale might say, sent chills down here spine. Nevertheless, Aubrey felt accomplished, as the spin instructor assured them that they had each burned over a thousand calories. As she left, she waved good-bye to the front desk girl.

"Bye Aubrey, I hope I see you soon!" exclaimed the front desk girl.

"Bye," Aubrey replied. *Was she implying that I won't return? How did she know my name? Why does she care if I come back?*

Nonetheless, the front desk girl was not going to ruin her mood. It was a New Year and Aubrey was a woman on a mission. She managed to get through an intense, one-hour spin class, her first workout in six months. Her new plan included six days of exercise; an enhancement to this year's New Year Resolution. That way, if she missed one or two days, she would still exercise four days. She also started her new diet, "20 Pounds in 20 Days," which was an aggressive juicing diet. Although Aubrey had tried this diet several times before, this time she was sure it would work. This was her year, nothing like last year or the year before. Aubrey sat in her car, which was littered with fast food wrappers, and stared into space.

Gosh, I am tired and starving. I know I started my diet today, but I have been good all day and work was stressful. I should go home and make juiced lemonade ... but since I burned a ton of calories I could pass by Tom's and get a smaller combo. Yeah, that's it. Just tonight. Tomorrow I'll be better. Plus, I deserve it. I trained hard today.

Aubrey proceeded to her favorite fast food place and ordered her usual meal. Although she had good intentions, since her workout was excruciating, she believed she had earned her meal. After a few hours of watching her favorite shows, Aubrey lay in bed and gazed at the ceiling.

What were those skinny girls talking about? Getting skinny isn't easy. It's been tough my whole life. What nerve they have saying that the biggest problem I have, they can do in a breeze. They probably have fast metabolisms or probably starve themselves.

Aubrey had battled her weight since college, and her recent divorce elevated the issue. For the past three years, since the divorce was finalized, she had tried many different weight loss methods. Everything from "Getting Shredded in 90 Days," funny shoes that are supposed to lift your butt, weird salt sprinkled on food, belts that shock you, ab contraptions, starvation cleanses, fat burners, and even a questionable vibrating stick! Shattered dreams were the only result.

"Beep ... Beep ... Beep... " Aubrey's alarm sounded. Each day, she hit the snooze button at least five times before she got up. As she began to move, she had a strange feeling. She was either dead or her body didn't function anymore. She started to realize that her body was feeling last night's workout. She smirked and thought, *Well, no pain, no gain, right?*

Aubrey scrambled to get ready for work (she was always running late), gulped her scheduled lemonade, and sped off to work. She was a junior executive at one of the top PR firms in the country. She had been there since graduating college, roughly ten years, and had worked her way up in the company.

"Good morning, Aubrey," welcomed her secretary.

"Oh, hey Carrie," replied Aubrey.

"You don't look well. Are you okay?"

"Hmm? Oh yeah, I'm fine, just hurting from my spin class. My butt is sore! Everything, and I mean everything, hurts. It even hurts when I go to the … I'll spare you the details," joked Aubrey. "But you know what they say, 'No pain, no gain.'"

"I guess," replied Carrie.

"What do you mean?"

"Well, one of my skinny friends said that exercise doesn't have to hurt," said Carrie. Carrie was a heavyset woman who had forty pounds to lose. She too had tried every fad diet and started each week with a new revolutionary diet. Oddly enough, she always seemed to be getting slightly bigger.

Aubrey didn't give the remark much thought as she commenced her work day. She read emails, took phone calls, and worked nonstop. A huge deadline was looming and Aubrey needed to complete an important presentation. Presentations for major clients placed added stress on Aubrey, and this was no exception. She got anxious whenever work escalated. As lunchtime approached, her mood began to lift. She looked forward to lunch. It was her time to escape the pressures of the day, to reward herself for all her hard work.

Oh, that's right, that stupid diet. Suddenly lunch seemed neither appealing nor rewarding. As Aubrey went to the break room to pick up her lemonade, she remembered that she hadn't told anybody about her latest diet. If she cheated, no one would judge her with their beady little eyes. She darted to her car and had lunch at her favorite Mexican restaurant.

Ahh, that was delicious. As she drove back to the office, horrible feelings of guilt haunted her. But when she arrived, she told that pesky little voice inside her head to shut up. Soon the work pressure resumed and Aubrey was back at it. Hours flew by and it was time to go home.

Should I go to the gym? I don't know; I'm kind of tired. It's been a long day. She contemplated going to the gym as she had on many occasions. Even accompanied with good intentions, she could somehow manage to talk herself out of exercising.

I know! I'll go double tomorrow! Aubrey skipped out to visit a different favorite fast food joint and ordered her favorite cheeseburger. *What a day.* After a few mind-numbing hours of her favorite shows, Aubrey crawled to bed.

The next day was the usual—another stressful episode. As Aubrey approached the gym after work, she remembered her promise to go double. That didn't happen, but Aubrey did manage to make it to spin class. Her body was very sore from the first class, and she left halfway through the class. On her way out, she bumped into the front desk girl.

"Aubrey, you made it back. Congrats! Are you done early?" questioned the front desk girl.

Embarrassed, Aubrey shifted her eyes, "Umm, I have an important presentation that I have to get ready for. You see, I can't stay the full hour. But at least I came in. It's better than nothing."

"Good for you. Keep it up! You'll get there soon enough," said the peppy front desk girl.

Whatever you skinny, little ... "Thank you," said Aubrey.

After her workout, Aubrey decided to continue her attempt at being healthy. Juicing was a wishful memory, but she grudgingly ordered a sandwich. There was little solace as she continued her commitment to try and shed her shameful, unwanted weight.

Who's This Skinny Guy Anyway?

Aubrey continued with her well-intentioned effort and haphazard approach to fitness. When she started her new program, she had planned for a lemonade juice cleanse, six days of working out, and no chocolate cake. As she ended her third week, however, she had completed one and a half days on the lemonade diet, a total of four workouts, and enjoyed three chocolate cakes. She stared at her office wall and slammed her head onto her desk. *I've had almost as many chocolate cakes as I had workouts! What's wrong with me? How come I can't stick to this? I'm such a failure. I should just give up and be fat, at least then I'll be happy.*

As she was moping, Carrie walked in.

"Oops, sorry Aubrey."

Aubrey's head rose with a saddened look and tears in her eyes. "It's okay, Carrie. Just sitting here sulking at my failures. Why can't I lose weight?"

"Well, I don't know. You look perfectly fine to me."

"You don't have to kid me, I know I'm overweight. I tried this time, I really tried. It's so freaking frustrating," said Aubrey.

"I know, I know ..." A long silence followed. "Well, have you tried that Mr. Skinny guy?" asked Carrie.

"Mr. Skinny? Who's that?"

"He's the trainer at the Total Body Project gym. My friend lost a ton of weight working with him. She swears he is the absolute best," said Carrie.

"I don't know. I don't really like trainers. I've had bad

experiences with them," she said.

"I think it's at least worth a shot. I heard his clients are 90% successful. The only problem is booking him," said Carrie.

"I don't know, we'll see. Thanks for listening to my whining, Carrie."

"Ha ha! No problem. We've all been there, trust me," she said as she shrugged.

After work, Aubrey dragged herself to the gym. Her eyes fixed on Mr. Skinny when she walked in. He was training his client, and although they were exercising, there seemed to be way too much talking going on.

That's odd. Why are they talking so much? She should be pumping iron. Well, whatever, time for spin class.

Aubrey made it through another challenging spin class. As she left, she cleverly stretched next to Mr. Skinny.

"Congrats, Lisa! I'm proud of you for losing twenty-five pounds! And I'm pumped for your first half marathon on Sunday! Can you believe six months ago you couldn't even run a mile? You have come a long way," cheered Mr. Skinny.

Mr. Skinny had a lean, athletic body, complete with a charismatic smile, but he seemed a little too happy for people.

"Thank you, Mr. Skinny. I never knew that at my age, I could accomplish such heights. I feel amazing!"

Mr. Skinny walked away with his client.

Hmm, I wonder. Could this Mr. Skinny character help me? I don't know. Ah, what the heck. She quickly gathered her stuff and ran to the front desk.

"Hi, Aubrey," said the front desk girl.

"Hi."

"How can I be of great service?"

Aubrey leaned over the counter and whispered, "What can you tell me about Mr. Skinny?"

The front desk girl smiled. "Let me guess. You want to train with him, right?"

"Well, maybe. How did you know?"

"Everybody wants to train with him. He's the best. He trained me," she said. The front desk girl was in outstanding shape. "Yeah, he trains all of the employees. He says he wants his staff to know and truly understand fitness. It makes our gym special."

"Does he work with other clients? Like gym members?" asked Aubrey.

"A few, but the ones he has, he's trained for years. I don't know if he's taking on new clients."

"Can you ask him?"

"Well, he's standing right behind you," she said as she pointed in his direction.

Aubrey turned around and smiled, "Hello, Mr. Skinny."

"Hi. I can see you ladies are having fun over here talking about me," he said, smiling. "Hopefully you were at least saying good things."

"Well, yes. I was wondering ... Can you, or... will you ..." she began asking.

"Train you?" he replied.

Aubrey nodded.

"That depends; how bad do you want it?" he asked.

"I want it very bad," she said.

"Are you willing to do everything I tell you to do?"

"Like what?" she responded.

"Like listen and learn everything I teach you?"

"Yup," said Aubrey.

"And," interjected Mr. Skinny.

"And?"

"Log your food, do your cardio, and listen with an open mind," he continued.

"You want me to log my food?" Aubrey responded with distaste. "Okay, I guess."

"Okay? Then maybe," he said and walked away.

Aubrey was puzzled and offended, but she chased after him anyway.

"Maybe? What does that mean?"

"Listen, Aubrey, correct? I've been doing this for fifteen years and if you're not fully committed, I am not going to waste your time or mine. I am not here to play games. You are either in or out. My reputation depends on the success of my clients and I take that personally. If you are not ready to commit, then don't."

Aubrey was taken aback by his approach. Here she was trying

to give the man business, but he didn't seem to want it.

"I know you've failed and been burned dozens of times. I am sorry for that. But if you're not serious, then I can't help you. I'm booked right now anyway; the earliest available appointment would be in two weeks and it's only temporary while one of my clients travels. Here's my number. If you decide to get serious, call me and I promise to try and help you as much as I can."

Aubrey took the card, and as she walked to her car, she replayed the sentence, "I promise to try and help you as much as I can." She felt secure; finally she would not be alone in this ordeal. She grabbed her phone, took a deep breath, and dialed.

"Hello, this is Mr. Skinny."

"I'm ready."

Get Me Skinny!!

What if he can't help me? I wonder if he is going to think I am too fat? What if I fail? What if ... What if? Aubrey was riled up. She was anxious about her first session with Mr. Skinny. His reputation as a no-nonsense straight shooter made her uneasy.

"Aubrey?"

"Yes, hello," Mr. Skinny's warm smile made her feel less uncomfortable.

"Are you ready? I'm super excited to get you going."

Wow! This guy is happy! I wonder if this is just an act. Oh well, at least it looks like he cares.

"Okay, Aubrey, today is simple. We are going to gather a little background information, take your picture, and learn about your goals. But most importantly, we are going to have fun! I am going to give you three homework assignments. Those homework assignments will help form the foundation for our mental fitness program. The mental programming aspect is as much if not more important than the physical one," explained Mr. Skinny as they walked through the gym.

What? We are not working out today? She was mentally prepped for an intense workout. When she realized Mr. Skinny would be asking her personal questions, she became embarrassed. She would be forced to answer! He might ask about her chocolate cake addiction. Not only that, but all she needed was another fat photo taken!

Mr. Skinny sensed Aubrey's tension. "Relax, Aubrey, today is *this is the heaviest I have ever been @ 211 lbs* *(5/30/13)*

the first day. Picture it like this: we'll draw a line in the sand and today will be the worst shape you will ever be in. From now on, each day, you will be in better shape. Every day will be a step forward, or maybe a step to the side, but never a step backwards. I believe in you."

20 weeks
Before
Nov 2nd

20
x 2 lbs/wk
40

Aubrey rolled her eyes, making sure Mr. Skinny didn't catch her; but it did feel nice to have someone believe in her.

They sat in his office, which was blanketed by incredible before-and-after photos. "Aubrey, what kind of fitness goals do you have?" asked Mr. Skinny.

"GET ME SKINNY!" Aubrey blurted. "Oops, I mean … you know …"

They both chuckled. "Ha ha, yes. I've never heard that before. And let me guess … Now, right?" replied Mr. Skinny. "Okay, it sounds like you want to lose weight."

Aubrey nodded.

"How much weight do you want to lose?"

"All of it," Aubrey smiled.

"I see," replied Mr. Skinny. This story sounded all too familiar. He had been a trainer for over fifteen years and it seemed like every client wanted to lose a significant amount of weight as soon as possible. This ill-fated strategy had major flaws. But he realized that exposing this truth early in the process could crush their hopes and motivation. "Okay, Aubrey, we are going to go as fast as possible. But honestly, my goal is to educate you and have you learn the most important principles in weight loss. When you learn these lessons, the education will stay with you for the rest of your life. Remember you are going to want to

12

be fit today, tomorrow, and forever. Fitness isn't a destination, it's a journey.

"What I need you to do is take this notebook. On one side, I want you to write down what you eat, including the time of day. I don't want you to worry about calories or anything yet. Also place a check mark each time you drink a glass of water. We are looking at behaviors, but I do want you to pay attention to that little voice in the back of your head. Right now, that little voice is quiet and subdued. We need to teach that voice how to get louder and move to the front of your mind. For now, just pay attention to it. On the other side of the notebook, you are going to write down Mr. Skinny's Power Analogies. These are fitness analogies that will help you understand fitness in simpler terms. Together they will form our MAD PLAN. I call it the MAD PLAN because each letter stands for a fitness pillar that is essential in our transformation."

Aubrey jotted down everything Mr. Skinny said. "This is a lot of stuff for working out," questioned Aubrey. *This guy is expensive, and all we're doing is taking notes, doing homework, and logging food? Are we even going to work out? I hope he knows what he's doing.*

"Correct. There are a lot of things you have to learn to get in shape. You need to understand why you are doing the elements in my program. Understanding the rationale is crucial to success," said Mr. Skinny. He had been successful with 90% of his clients. If Aubrey listened, she would enjoy the same success.

"Now, before I give you your homework, I need you to be real with me," lectured Mr. Skinny.

Aubrey grew nervous, but nodded in agreement.

"The most important element in any program is to first accept responsibility for your decisions and consequent actions. This is nonnegotiable. If you cannot commit to this, then we stop here. I will be of no use to you. But if you can commit to this simple but powerful philosophy, you will enjoy a life with the body you have always dreamt of. Aubrey, can you take full responsibility for your actions?"

Aubrey turned and stared into one of the giant mirrors.

Aubrey pondered the question. This was a new and profound concept. She flashed back to her previous weight loss attempts when she had blamed the stupid ab device, the dreaded starvation diet, the weird movie star workouts, the saboteurs offering her junk food, and those sweet Girl Scout cookie pushers. She had blamed everyone and everything except herself.

"Aubrey?" Mr. Skinny interjected.

"Huh? I mean yes. I can," Aubrey snapped back.

"Good. I promise this is one of the best decisions you will ever make. I am proud of you already. It takes immense courage to come talk to me about receiving help. You are on your way to success and I want you to know that I am here for you. I will always be here for you. Today, tomorrow, and long after our sessions are done. Now smile and say 'Cheese,' and remember, say it, don't eat it," joked Mr. Skinny.

Aubrey laughed. "I love cheese," she said as she gave a smile. "Cheeese."

"Thank you, Mr. Skinny. That means a lot to me," replied Aubrey. She felt better and felt fortunate for the opportunity to work with Mr. Skinny—her first real partner in this journey.

Mr. Skinny handed Aubrey her first homework assignment and instructed her to open her notebook for her first analogy.

"You see, Aubrey, this journey is like traveling through a strange forest. You don't know the exact way or how far or how treacherous the quest will be. The true perils of the forest lie in the unknown. How can you survive alone? I, on the other hand, have been through the forest many times. I have safely traversed the difficult paths with a variety of people, taking special note of each of their strengths and providing an appropriate course. Not only can I map the route, I also know the fastest, safest, and most secure way. So listen intently, follow closely, and enjoy the fruits of success."

Aubrey was off! She felt great about her first day with Mr. Skinny. Their next appointment was in a week, but she had homework to complete. She wrote down her food and tried to listen to that little voice in the back of her head. *Okay, little voice don't fail me now.*

What in the World Is a Calorie?

> Congratulations and welcome to the rest of your life! Your first task is to learn as much as possible about the relationship between a calorie and the Law of Conservation of Energy.

Aubrey read her first homework assignment in her notebook and began doing research on the subjects.

> Calorie: a unit of energy, defined as the amount of energy required to raise the temperature of 1 gram of water 1 degree Celsius

> Law of Conservation of Energy: Energy cannot be created nor destroyed.

> One pound is equal to 3,500 calories.

As Aubrey wrote down these facts, she began to wonder about the relationship between food and exercise. *It seems like the energy I take in, or calories, and the energy I burn, or calories out, are the same. Could this be right? This seems too simple. This can't be right. Mr. Skinny will clear this up.*

She logged her food, including the times, for the rest of the week. The muffled voice in her head would try to stop Aubrey from bad choices, but it was powerless against Aubrey's reasoning. Even the guilty feelings didn't alter Aubrey's behavior, but she did attempt to be more mindful of her food decisions as she knew Mr. Skinny would review her log.

Aubrey arrived the next week complete with her food log and homework assignment ready for her workout.

"Welcome back, Aubrey," Mr. Skinny said as he shook her hand.

"Oh, hey. How are you?"

"I am fantastic; another day living my dream," replied Mr. Skinny. His suspicious enthusiasm was radiating. "Okay, let's have a look."

Mr. Skinny studied Aubrey's food log and made notes. He placed happy faces next to the good choices and circled all of the junk food. He also noted the spacing between the meals. "Okay, it doesn't look too bad."

Aubrey was shocked, "Really?"

"For your first week, I mean. All I was looking for was honesty, responsibility, and timing of meals. You are being honest and accepting responsibility."

"Did I make too many bad choices?" Aubrey asked.

"Well, yes," replied Mr. Skinny with a half smile.

"You see, Aubrey, it's like a choice scale. You need to analyze all of your choices for the past year on this imaginary balance scale. On the left side you have all the year's bad choices, and on the right side you have all the good choices. In your particular case, you are skewed to the left. Your balance has more bad choices than good ones. As you begin to positively move forward, the scales will tilt in your favor. Slowly but surely, you will add more good choices and the balance will tilt toward the middle. When the scale is balanced, you will have just as many good choices as bad choices. But to make real progress, you need more good choices. You need to be good a lot longer than you were bad."

Aubrey wrote down her second analogy. "Now, let's look back

and remember that little voice inside your head. Remember that guy?" continued Mr. Skinny.

"Yeah, I heard him, but I just ignored him. You know, he can be really annoying," replied Aubrey.

Mr. Skinny chuckled, "Yeah, I know how you feel. But you need to empower that voice to help you make better decisions. Did you drink any water?"

Aubrey was embarrassed and shook her head, "I was busy at work and forgot."

"Aubrey, water is very important. Did you know that when we are thirsty our mind interprets it as hunger?"

"Really?"

"Water is an easy way to help you feel full. That way, you are less likely to make bad decisions. This is easy and you have to do it. Got it?" scolded Mr. Skinny.

"Yes, more water. Got it," nodded Aubrey.

"I also noted where I think another small meal should go. You don't want too much time to lapse between meals. And by meals, I mean every time you eat, even snacks. You want to eat on a consistent basis. The rationale is simple. When you go too long between meals, more than five or six hours, your body becomes confused and feels like it is not going to eat again for another five or six hours. This causes a chemical reaction in your brain that triggers a craving of fattier foods. Your body craves fattier foods because they contain more stored energy."

"Oh, wow. I didn't know that," replied Aubrey. She only ate twice per day, usually lunch and dinner, but her life was chaotic. She wondered where she would find time for breakfast and snacks. "What can I eat for snacks?"

"You want to eat every three to four hours. When it's time for a small snack, it can be anything healthy around two hundred calories. An apple, orange, meal-replacement bar, or cheese stick would work. The key is consistent, small meals," explained Mr. Skinny.

"You see, Aubrey, it's like Thanksgiving dinner. We know it as a day to not only feast, but to gorge. To let loose and eat anything and everything our little hearts desire. Most people wait the whole day, refusing to eat until dinner, and end up starving themselves. They starve themselves with one intention: when the special dinner arrives in their tummy, it will have the taste of legends. Now, let's take the same meal, spectacular and everything. What happens if you eat an apple right before? What happens to the legendary taste, the meal fit for kings? It doesn't taste the same, does it? It tastes ordinary. Does that strike you as odd? The actual food composition hasn't changed one bit. The difference is how our mind interprets the food. It's fascinating."

Aubrey knew she was guilty of behaving that exact way. If she ate right before, she somehow spoiled her dinner. It didn't taste the same. She hadn't thought about it in that particular fashion.

"You are on the right path, Aubrey. Congratulations," said Mr. Skinny. "Now, let's take a look at your research." Aubrey pulled out her information.

"Now, what do you think all this science stuff means?" questioned Mr. Skinny.

Aubrey was surprised. "I thought you were going to answer that," she replied.

Mr. Skinny smiled. "Well, I already know what it means. I want to know what you think."

Aubrey wasn't sure how to respond. She stood in silence.

"Aubrey, you told me that you are a junior executive at your firm, correct?"

Aubrey nodded.

"You don't get to positions like yours by not thinking. I want you to think about this and give me the correct interpretation," said Mr. Skinny in a stern voice.

Aubrey felt challenged and wanted to respond. She studied her notes and said, "Well, according to the Law of Conservation of Energy, energy cannot be created nor can it be destroyed. Energy is measured in terms of calories. One pound is equal to thirty-five hundred calories; therefore, to lose one pound, I need to burn thirty-five hundred calories."

1 lb = 3500 calories

"Yes, that's correct. What else?"

What else? What is this guy talking about? Aubrey scratched her head.

"How does someone lose or gain weight?" said Mr. Skinny.

"Ah! Well, if I eat more than I burn, I will gain weight. If I eat the same calories as I burn, my weight will stay the same. If I eat fewer calories and burn more calories, I will lose weight! BAM!!" exclaimed Aubrey. "Wait, that's it?!"

"Actually, when it comes to weight loss, this is the only equation you need to understand. Understand and master," lectured Mr. Skinny.

"That's it? Really?"

"That's it! I promise you, that's it. Nothing more," explained Mr. Skinny.

"So, you're telling me all I have to do is be in a caloric deficit to lose weight? What about carbs, proteins, sugars, organic, and all that stuff I keep hearing about?"

"Well, that's wrong ... Ha ha! Okay, well, not exactly. Aubrey, for the time being, all you need to do is worry about the energy balance in your body. You have to take in fewer calories than you burn. You need to increase activities like walking, running, exercising, cardio, and resistance training; in essence, increase your energy out. At the same time, you have to decrease your energy intake, or the calories from the food you eat. For our purposes, the actual breakdown of the macronutrients, fats, carbs, and proteins, are not going to matter. I mean, obviously you don't want to have all fat, but your weight loss is going to boil down to this energy relation. You have to understand it and you have to master it; eat less and move more. Sounds simple, right?"

Aubrey smiled and nodded.

"Well ... not exactly," interjected Mr. Skinny. "Doesn't this relationship sound familiar? Who wants to be rich?" Aubrey raised her hand. "Everyone always yells 'Me, me, me!' Easy enough: earn more and spend less. We all understand the basic principle well. The problem lies in the execution," explained Mr. Skinny.

"You see, Aubrey, managing calories is like managing money. If you want to lose weight, burn more calories than you eat. If you want to be rich, make more money than you spend. Pretty simple, huh? The difference is that with money you have precise vision. When you are the beneficiary of a raise or a gift, you know exact numbers. If you overspend money, you see your account balance drop. Unfortunately, this isn't the case with food. Without being able to see your food balance, you are forced to guess. You have to guess at how many calories you take in and how many calories you burn. Sadly, you usually guess in your own selfish favor."

Aubrey nodded in amazement. The blurry world of fitness was starting to come into focus. She was eager to start applying this newfound information.

Mr. Skinny continued, "Aubrey, the beauty in this plan is the simplicity. We all understand budgeting in monetary terms and soon you will learn how to manage a budget in caloric terms. But the magic sauce for weight loss lies in the execution. The real problem is in you and your stifled little voice. Right now, your voice is quiet, passive, and helpless. We need to train that voice to become a powerful force in your decision making. It is not so much what you do, but rather, the real discovery is to tackle why you do."

Aubrey was floored; this Mr. Skinny guy had broken down the science into easy, understandable terms.

"Make sense?" asked Mr. Skinny.

"Completely."

They proceeded to go over a few stretches and light cardio for the workout.

"Okay, for your next homework assignment, I am going to have you meet a close friend of mine. Let him know that I sent you and remember to take full responsibility for your choices."

Paging Dr. M

"Good morning, Aubrey," welcomed Carrie.

"And what a wonderful morning it is!" replied Aubrey.

"Wow! You're in a good mood. How's the training going? Is it intense? I heard he's brutal."

"It's fantastic, and honestly, the workouts haven't been too hard ... they haven't felt like workouts at all," replied Aubrey.

Carrie gave her a weird expression and answered the ringing phone. "Blakely and Associates, this is Carrie, how may I direct your call? ... Okay, she just stepped in. Can I place you on hold? Thank you ... Aubrey, it's for you. It's a Dr. M."

"Hello?" answered Aubrey.

"Hi, Aubrey, this is Dr. M. I am returning your call. My secretary said you are a friend of Mr. Skinny."

"Yes, that is correct. He is my personal trainer," replied Aubrey.

"Congratulations, that is wonderful news. Mr. Skinny was also my trainer. He helped me lose eighty pounds and helped me to restructure the way I do my job. I'm a cardiologist at the hospital," said Dr. M.

Aubrey was shocked that Mr. Skinny had assigned her to see a cardiologist. She had been diagnosed as a pre-diabetic with high cholesterol and blood pressure. Hospitals frightened her.

"How does tomorrow at noon sound?" asked Dr. M.

"That should work, thank you," replied Aubrey.

"Perfect, I'll have my nurse send you all the details. I need to return to surgery."

This made Aubrey more nervous. Hospitals scared her, but surgeries really scared her.

The next day, Aubrey arrived at the hospital filled with even more fear. When she checked in she learned that Dr. M worked in emergency care. *Great, just great,* she thought.

"Aubrey?"

"Yes," nodded Aubrey.

"Hi, I'm Dr. M. It is a pleasure to meet you. First off, let me congratulate you on your choice to get in shape. I am very proud of you," said Dr. M.

This struck Aubrey as odd. *Why would he care about me?* Dr. M was a tall, dark and slender man in his early forties. He wore glasses and spoke with a slight Spanish accent. They exchanged pleasantries and Dr. M sent Aubrey to prep for surgery.

"Not me!" she shouted.

"No, Aubrey, of course not you. You are going to observe a heart surgery. We are going to perform a surgery on a patient whose BIGGER BURN has failed," assured Dr. M.

Aubrey wasn't sure what he meant, but she was happy to learn that the procedure wasn't meant for her. As she prepared for surgery, she thought, *Wow, this is nerve-racking. My doctor warned me of all the heart trouble I could have if I don't watch my weight. I hate being in here; it feels too real.*

"Paging Dr. M. Dr. M to the operating room," yelled a voice over the intercom.

Both Dr. M. and Aubrey were in scrubs and ready for surgery. As they walked toward the operating room, Dr. M prepped her.

"Aubrey, we are going to encounter a patient whose BIGGER BURN has failed. Consequently, we need to perform bypass surgery on his heart for him to live. This is one of the last chances he has to survive. We need to perform the surgery and try to reinstall his new BIGGER BURN. If we are successful, he has a chance. If we fail, unfortunately, there is no chance," said Dr. M.

They rushed into the operating room and a large man lay with his chest wide open. Aubrey watched in horror and disbelief as the medical team performed heart surgery. *I can't believe this is what happens to people. People talk about this all the time, but to actually stand here and watch such a procedure is eye-opening. If I don't turn my life around, this is where I'll end up. I cannot let this happen to me.*

The surgery continued for several hours and Aubrey watched somberly. When it was over, Dr. M left the operating room with Aubrey.

"Aubrey, did you see what happened?"

"Yes, you performed heart surgery."

"Yes, but do you know why?" asked Dr. M.

"Because his heart was in trouble," answered Aubrey.

"Well, that's partially correct," said Dr. M. "Aubrey, follow me to the BIGGER BURN room."

Uh, oh. Aubrey thought. *What the heck was the BIGGER BURN room? Was it more frightening than the operating room?* They marched to a room on the other side of the hospital. As they stepped in, Aubrey noticed a number of overweight patients. *What in the world is going on in this room?*

"Have a seat, Aubrey," said Dr. M as he handed her a questionnaire. "Please fill this out and I'll be right with you."

Aubrey looked at the questionnaire and began to fill it out. It asked for standard background information and it contained interesting questions pertaining to her goals: *5/30/13*

How much weight do you need to lose? *70 lbs*

How much weight do you want to lose? *80 lbs*

Why? *To be healthy & for my clothes to fit better*

No, really? Why? *To look and feel sexy. To be able to get into a size 8* *Best feeling ever.*

That's interesting, Aubrey thought. *These questions are redundant. And why is there so much room to answer?*

When Aubrey finished filling out the form, she flipped over the clipboard, which had a few fun facts about the BIGGER BURN room.

Did you know?

The BIGGER BURN room was founded 15 years ago by Dr. M.

90% of his patients are successful with their weight loss goal.

Most patients who lose the weight never gain it back.

Over 68% of the U.S. is overweight, with 34% considered obese.

Over 7 million people per year die of heart disease.

Heart disease is the #1 killer in the U.S.

Wow, this is interesting, Aubrey thought.

"Aubrey?" asked the nurse.

"That's me," replied Aubrey.

"The doctor will see you now."

Aubrey walked in and sat in a bizarre room. She was surrounded by quotes, before-and-after pictures, testimonials, and inspiring messages.

Dr. M sat gazing outside his large window; he turned his ominous chair around.

"Aubrey, I understand that you were sent to me by Mr. Skinny. I am delighted to help you. I am sure he explained to you the power of honesty, choice, and responsibility," continued Dr. M.

Aubrey nodded.

"Okay, let's look at your answers," he said as he shook his head.

"This just isn't going to do. No, no, no." Dr. M accelerated his head shaking.

Aubrey froze; her heart began to race. *What is Dr. M talking about? Why isn't this going to work? Am I in trouble? What is going on?*

"I mean, your reasons are okay, Aubrey," started Dr. M. "But what we are searching for is the 'why,' or, as we like to call it, the 'BIGGER BURN.'"

Aubrey had written down: "I just want to be healthy," and "so I can fit into my old clothes."

Dr. M took off his glasses and said, "I cannot emphasize enough how important this is. Do you remember the operating room?"

Aubrey nodded.

"That, Aubrey, was Mr. Taylor. He fell into our ten percent. These are the patients whose BIGGER BURN has failed them. When our BIGGER BURN fails, it means that nothing else will work. At this point, lifesaving heart surgery will, sadly, only partially help."

"Only partially?"

"Yes, Aubrey. Since he never established a powerful enough BIGGER BURN, he failed and so did his heart. And you know what?" asked Dr. M.

"What?"

"The saddest part is that even after quadruple bypass surgery, it will only buy him time. Soon after the surgery, he will forget what he had to endure, and the same old hideous habits that caused him the original heart trouble will rear its ugly head."

Aubrey was shocked and astonished at this revelation. She considered herself overweight, but hoped that she would get it under control before it was too late.

"That's how important your BIGGER BURN is, Aubrey. This compelling reason will be your north star, your guiding light, your moral compass—the 'why.' The BIGGER BURN is the reason you will be successful this time. But this is a question only you can answer. It is a deep truth that has a significant meaning and emotion associated. You know you have the right BIGGER BURN when it feels good but also makes you vulnerable when expressed. The BIGGER BURN has to be personal and meaningful in order for progress to occur.

"I realize that this is hard to express, because it opens you up emotionally. Most of us are fearful of being vulnerable. We give surface answers that do not allow for us to progress," said Dr. M. "Most of us don't want to expose our vulnerability, so when we're out with friends and they inevitably ask you, 'Why are you doing this?' you pause, and then give the typical, meaningless answer, 'Well, I just want to lose a couple pounds,' or 'I just want to be healthy,' or blah, blah, blah. That is a cool, politically correct answer, and you can keep that for social interactions. But for you to be successful now, you are going to have to do better. You need a cause that will either move you toward gain or away from pain. You need to find that deep, touching, and magical spark to ignite a fire of burning desire. When you find this, you will be amazed at how you can move mountains. How you will feel unstoppable, how it will feel like it was meant to be. When you find that deep, inner layer of powerful motivation, the world will feel like it is at your fingertips and you can accomplish anything."

Aubrey could feel his passion and was beginning to be moved. She had never tried to pinpoint such a deep feeling, refusing to even acknowledge the emotion for fear of judgment. Also, failing would hurt even more with her true reason out in the open. There was a long silence between the two. Both knew that this was a moment that would change Aubrey's life forever.

"Well ..." Aubrey started; she hesitated and was nervous about telling a stranger her deepest desires.

Dr. M noticed her inner turmoil and said, "Let's begin by being honest with me. Give me the real reason, and I mean I want the real reason. It can be a variety of reasons. The key element in this process is that I need to find out if you are a 'move toward gain' or 'away from pain' type of person. Your particular BIGGER BURN will fall into one of these two categories. Whichever category you fall into doesn't matter; what matters is the reason. It must be filled with burning emotion, passion, and a yearning desire. It has to raise the hairs on the back of your neck; it has to make you uncomfortable; it has to make you jump. In short, it has to be filled with craze, good or bad. Make it touching and powerful. Here are a few examples of the BIGGER BURNS that my patients have used in the past. Now, keep in mind that these are reasons that we don't go out and advertise. We hold these reasons close to the vest. They are powerful and if misused can cause significant hurt:

'Honestly, I'm just tired of looking and feeling fat. I don't like it and it doesn't make me feel good.'

'Being overweight makes me feel ugly.'

'I never want to be in a bathing suit.'

'I want to walk into a meeting without everyone staring at me. I am afraid of what they are thinking.'

'I am sick and tired of my husband staring at other women.'

'For once in my life, I want to look hot!'

'I have a destination beach wedding coming and I don't want to feel embarrassed.'

'I hate feeling insecure.'

'I hate how my thighs touch.'

'My wedding is coming up and we all know pictures are forever. I want to be at my best for this special moment in my life.'

'I was watching a video filmed at work and I saw a fat guy in the background. I thought to myself, Wow, look at chubs. That chubs turned out to be me. I didn't realize I had gotten so big.'

'I need to find a partner in life, and without confidence, I don't have a chance.'

"These are a few of the stories of BIGGER BURNS, and as I tell them to you, I can vividly recall the emotion inside each one of my patients. It either hurt badly or it felt good, but the most important element was that they felt. I knew as soon as we had this information we would be able to accomplish anything. Now, let's stop and search inside of you. What we are looking for here is honesty, the real reason, the BIGGER BURN, the thought you can always use to center you. This image has to be ingrained in your mind. You have to feel it in every inch of your body. It has to burn to your core."

Aubrey sat for a moment. Words began to creep out of her mouth.

"Ahh, not for me, Aubrey. I want you to go home, think about this, and write down your BIGGER BURN. Always carry it with you, and when you are faced with a choice or you feel your goals are being compromised, reach in your pocket and touch it. You will feel invigorated, recharged, and closer to your goal."

Aubrey nodded and said, "Thank you so much Dr. M, you have no idea how much you have helped me."

"My pleasure, Aubrey. I am here to help and share the gift of fitness, Dr. Motivacion, at your service." A giant smile complete with sparking eyes arose from his face.

"Ahh, of course," Aubrey smiled.

Aubrey left the hospital oozing with excitement. She had an idea about what her BIGGER BURN was, but she wasn't one hundred percent sure.

As fate would have it, that night, Aubrey had a terrible nightmare that woke her. Covered in a cold sweat, she took out a piece of paper and wrote down her BIGGER BURN. *Aha! This is it! This is really it!*

Oh, No!! What Is This?

When Aubrey met with Mr. Skinny again, he checked her food log and asked about cardio, stretching, and vitamins. He smiled and said, "Okay, Aubrey, let me see it."

Aubrey took out a folded up note and handed it over.

"Yes! Powerful—a perfect BIGGER BURN," smiled Mr. Skinny. "This will work. This will work."

Aubrey was thrilled even though it was embarrassing to let out such deep emotions. It felt liberating and it felt right. She trusted Mr. Skinny and knew he had her best intentions at heart. After a light workout, Aubrey was on her way home.

She felt accomplished. Her clothes were beginning to fit a little looser. As she walked into her office, she had an extra pep in her step. *This is working, really working*, she thought.

"You're looking lean, Aubrey. Have you lost some weight?" asked Carrie.

"Maybe? I think so, but I don't get measured till next week," replied Aubrey.

"That's great news. Sounds like you're on it. Happy hour Friday night?"

Aubrey paused and said, "Sure, why not? I'm doing great and I'm getting skinny. Let's do it!"

Aubrey was ecstatic; although it was only a subtle change, for others to notice, it made all the difference in the world. The motivation, the food log, Mr. Skinny—it was all working! Aubrey felt on top of the world.

Then she went home and opened her mail.

Oh no, what is this? Aubrey ripped opened a letter. It was from the IRS; they wanted to see her immediately. She broke into a cold sweat and began to panic. *I thought I paid my taxes? Did they find out about those iffy donations? Oh, this can't be good.* She was in full panic mode. The document said to meet with an auditor that Friday at the local office.

Aubrey hardly slept that night as the audit raced through her mind. She tried to remember every single item that was on her report. *I think I did everything right? What could they possibly want with me? I always make sure to turn in my taxes on time. I double and triple-check everything. Oh, well. I guess, I'll just see what happens.*

That Friday, Aubrey walked into the IRS office, took a number, and sat down. Around the room, people looked eerily similar to the operating room at the hospital, complete with pained looks on their faces. She began to agonize.

"Aubrey?" said the auditor.

"Yes, that's me," replied Aubrey.

"Hi, follow me," said the auditor. They walked into a separate office, with a lone desk and two chairs. He sat in front of her and asked, "Now, Aubrey, do you know why you are here?"

"No," replied Aubrey quivering.

The auditor noticed her tension and said, "Oh, I'm sorry. Let me introduce myself. My name is Miyagi Akira and I am a senior accountant. But more importantly, I am a friend of Mr. Skinny." A huge sigh of relief flashed across Aubrey's face.

"Oh wow, did he call you to scare me? Because you sure did a good job," Aubrey said.

"Oh, I'm sorry about that. But that was intentional. It was meant for dramatic effect. You see, my job is to teach you about accountability." He took out Aubrey's taxes from the past few years and said, "You have done a tidy job reporting your taxes. You've been complete and thorough."

Aubrey smiled.

"You never had anything to worry about, yet you felt anxious at the mere thought of an examination."

"Yeah, why is that?"

"Well, Aubrey, the funny thing about humans is that we don't do things if people aren't going to check them," explained Miyagi.

Aubrey scratched her head.

"You complete your taxes every year because you know they will be checked and you will be held accountable. There are also legal consequences that help motivate you. Accountability is central to success in people as it is in any organization. This is the primary reason that colleges, therapists, nutritionists, and trainers are successful. They install a fabricated deadline for you to complete a specific project. You see, most of us lack the discipline to complete the task on our own. We need external deadlines to ensure projects get done."

Aubrey nodded.

"You see, Aubrey, weight loss is like that ten-page paper that you had due in college. Remember those good old college days when you looked at the syllabus and thought, 'That's not due till week seven, I have plenty of time'? And there you found yourself, trying to print your paper minutes before it was due. But, you got it done. Why? Because it was being collected. You were being held accountable. For weight loss, this 'paper' you have to turn in gets collected when? Never. So what happens? You procrastinate and don't get it done. And if you make horrible nutrition choices, the 'paper' gets longer. You forget to work on it, and you get the point. Nothing happens. With no one there to check your progress, you can only hold yourself accountable, which might not be a good thing."

Aubrey took out her notebook. *He's right, whenever I set my own goals, I don't want to tell anybody. That way, if I fail, people can't judge me. And if I cheat, I tell myself, "Well, maybe not by February but by March for sure."*

"It is wise to collaborate with Mr. Skinny," continued Miyagi. "But, what will happen when Mr. Skinny isn't there? Or what about those who aren't fortunate enough to be able to afford a personal trainer? What then?"

"I, I don't know ... I am not sure," replied Aubrey. She was perplexed. *He's right, how can I do this without anyone's help? Mr. Skinny is my fitness accountant for now, but what about after?* This troubled her.

"It's simple, Aubrey," continued Miyagi. "There are many ways to make this work. But in my professional opinion, the most successful route is to form your own Accountability Alliance."

"A what?"

"An Accountability Alliance. In order for you to have any chance of making lasting behavior changes, you will need the help of those closest to you," said Miyagi.

Aubrey raised her eyebrows.

"Now, this can be a treacherous area to navigate. You might get moody, you might snap back, and you might feel judged," explained Miyagi.

"I know, I am scared of failing in the eyes of others," admitted Aubrey.

"Well, tough ... Do you really want to change? Take a long, hard look at those around you. Find one person at home, one person at work, and one close friend," said Miyagi. "Write down the names of your Accountability Alliance, those who will help you achieve your goal. Without a strong support team, you have no chance of succeeding. They need to know your BIGGER BURN and understand its importance. If they truly understand, you will be surprised by how helpful they will be. It's wonderful. They will help you in many ways, but be prepared," warned Miyagi.

"Okay," Aubrey said.

"No," Miyagi stopped her. "I mean really be prepared. When you appoint others to provide accountability, be ready. If you cheat, or even think about cheating, in front of them, you will receive dirty, shameful looks. This is a tough pill to swallow; if you cheat around them, you will feel tremendous guilt. It's one thing to let yourself down, but to let others down is another."

"Oh, I see. More eyes to help keep me on track," explained Aubrey.

"Exactly, Aubrey. You need them. You will benefit from the added strength and accountability. By leveraging those that are closest to you, you make the task of one the task of the whole," expressed Miyagi.

"You see, Aubrey, it's like the stick story. Let's say you are in the woods gathering sticks. One stick is easy to break; but if you pick up another similar stick and try to break them together, the sticks are more resilient. You pick up a third stick and even more strength is added. The sticks together are stronger than any stick individually."

"That sounds like a clever way to add more accountability without adding more work. I know the perfect people for my team!" exclaimed Aubrey. She was energized at this new opportunity. Making her weight loss everyone's task would help.

"Thank you so much for your help, Miyagi," said Aubrey.

"Well, don't thank me yet. I will get all the thanks I need when you reach your goal. I am happy for you; I believe in my heart that you will be successful. I know how important accountability is, and I believe you now know how important it is too. It has been my pleasure, Aubrey," said Miyagi.

As Aubrey left, she felt her phone vibrating in her purse.

"Hey, Carrie!" answered Aubrey.

"It's Friday girl! Happy hour time! Are you ready?"

"Yeah, just finishing up at the IRS. Long story, I'll tell you later. Just need to run home and change. I'll meet you guys there," said Aubrey.

"Perfect, see you in a bit," responded Carrie.

The girls liked to hang out at a local bar by their office. Their happy hours consisted of the usual appetizers and drinks.

"Another round!" shouted Carrie.

Aubrey could hear Carrie across the bar as she strolled in. She was apprehensive about attending happy hour. *I guess the girls started early*, she thought. *I mean, Mr. Skinny didn't say I couldn't attend happy hour. I'll be good, or just not as bad.* A slick smile emerged from Aubrey's face. As she muscled her way through the crowd, she caught a glimpse of her ex-husband.

No, that can't be him! It had been years and many pounds since she had seen him. She was embarrassed and abruptly changed paths. She ran to the bathroom to hide. *What is he doing here? He cannot see me like this! Ugh, I hate this. I am never coming back here again! Never!*

Aubrey joined the girls when the coast was clear. Without saying a word to the girls, she yelled, "Waiter, one of everything and shots, shots, lots of shots ... and on the double!"

You Will Fall ... Get Up!

"Hello, Aubrey. So, anything exciting happen?" said Mr. Skinny with a smirk.

Aubrey paused.

"Yeah ... thanks for the IRS summons," said Aubrey as she walked on the treadmill. She wrestled whether to tell Mr. Skinny about her drunken rage.

"Oops, yeah I know. I'm sorry about that. It is only meant to strike a chord," he replied.

"Yeah, trust me. I know. Not the chord I wanted, but I got the message loud and clear," said Aubrey.

"So, have you decided?"

"Decided what?" answered Aubrey.

"The three people for your Accountability Alliance."

"Oh that. Actually, yes; it was pretty easy to decide. Well, first of all you," she said, smiling. Mr. Skinny smiled and nodded. "Then Carrie, a girl from my work, and my sister Sarah."

"I think those are fine choices," he said and patted her on the back.

"Working as a team provides you the best chance of succeeding. Now, when you ask Carrie and Sarah to help, you must explain to them the significance of your BIGGER BURN. They need to feel your emotion, understand the severity, and realize the importance of accountability. Let them know that you might be moody and at times you might not like them, but that their support and presence will make all the difference in the world. And don't forget to thank them for being on your team."

"Really? I have to do all that?"

"Well, do you want to be successful?" Mr. Skinny asked. "If you speak with passion and conviction, they will understand the gravity of and respect your decision. In most cases, the people that care most about us want to see us succeed. Most of the time, they are the same ones attending our food dilemma episodes. But if they are on your team, armed with knowledge of your BIGGER BURN, and recognize your desire, they will be an invaluable asset. Our loved ones want to see us happy and they want to see us thrive. Luckily for us, if we need their help, we just need to ask."

Aubrey paused. *That's a great point,* she thought. *Every time I start a diet or a new workout program and tell someone about it, I joke, "Well, we'll see how long I keep this up." I laugh to mask the pain and keep the mood light, but sadly to also avoid facing the ugly truth of yet another failed attempt.*

"Okay, sir. Will do," agreed Aubrey.

"Great job today, Aubrey. That's it for today."

Aubrey grabbed Mr. Skinny, "Wait, listen. I have to tell you something."

Mr. Skinny tilted his head.

"I, I failed," said Aubrey with a look of disgust.

"How bad?"

"Real bad," she said. She looked down.

"Oh, I see," he said and turned away.

"Are you mad at me?"

"No, Aubrey, I could never be mad at you. But I don't want you to be reckless with your body anymore. Please have the respect to treat your body like it deserves to be treated. Remember, you only get one. I'm not mad, but I am disappointed."

"Great, that's like ten times worse. I feel awful. Why do I sabotage myself? Why?" Aubrey looked toward the sky.

"Hey listen, relax," Mr. Skinny said. "You made a mistake; it happens. But you need to learn from it. I wish you would have stuck to your program, but you made a mistake. It's spilled milk; let it go. You will make mistakes, but don't let them change your entire attitude. You screwed up. You will fall, but I need you to get up. Today is a new day. Be great today."

Aubrey sobbed.

"You see, Aubrey, it's like trying to dig a hole. Picture a mountain of sand, which represents all the calories that you have overeaten throughout the years. For you to succeed, you need a hole in that mountain of sand. Better get to digging. You grab your small shovel and work diligently to dig a deep hole. Digging, digging, day in and day out, working laboriously, covered in sweat through fall, winter, and spring. You pause to take a break and leave your hole unattended. A dump truck zooms in and drops a load of sand into your hole! That momentary lapse in judgment cost you your countless hours of digging in a matter of seconds. Mistakes are setbacks and are a part of life, but you must learn from them. You may want to give up, but you still need to dig. And dig a lot. You can't give up. You have no other choice."

"I'm sorry, I understand," said Aubrey as she departed.

Tomorrow is a new day. Today was difficult, but tomorrow will be better. These thoughts offered some comfort as Aubrey lay to rest for the evening.

"Good morning, Aubrey," welcomed Carrie.

"Good morning, Carrie. How are you today?"

"Ahh, you know, it's hump day, so blah," said Carrie. They shared a laugh.

"Listen, can you come into my office when you have a chance?"

"Is everything okay? Did he find out? Was he mad?" worried Carrie.

"Oh, yes, yes. Actually, it somehow worked out with Mr. Skinny. Listen, I want to ask for help on a special project."

"Oh really? Sure. Give me five minutes and I'll be right in." Carrie said.

Aubrey waited in her office.

"What a crazy night! Okay, how can I help?" said Carrie as she sat down.

Aubrey ignored her first comment, "Well, you have known me for about ten years. And you have seen me gain weight, lose some, and gain more."

"Well, we've all gained weight and I think you look gre-"

"And that's exactly it," Aubrey said, cutting her off.

"I am not happy where I am, and I need your help," said Aubrey.

"I am not sure what you mean," replied Carrie.

Aubrey reached in her pocket and handed Carrie her BIGGER BURN. Carrie read the small, wrinkled paper and began to tear up.

"I had no idea you felt this way," said Carrie.

"Do you see why I need your help?" Aubrey looked into Carrie's eyes.

Carrie nodded.

"This is important to me, and I need your help in holding me accountable. And I need your support. I can't do this without you," Aubrey said.

Carrie whipped around the desk and gave Aubrey a warm hug.

"I promise to help you as much as I can."

"Even if I kick and scream?" asked Aubrey.

Carrie smiled, "Even if you kick and scream."

"Thank you, Carrie. That means the world to me."

That went better than I thought. I already feel stronger. Now I just need to talk to my sister and I'll be set! Aubrey's wounded confidence was slowly healing.

The Little Voice

Mr. Skinny's workouts began to pick up steam, getting more advanced, and Aubrey started to lose a little more weight. The weight loss was happening, slowly but happening. Aubrey wanted it faster, but Mr. Skinny stressed to her that the real work was training her little voice. Her inner voice would establish the foundation for her success.

"You keep talking about this little voice. What do you mean?" Aubrey asked during a set of squats.

"Your little voice is getting louder," replied Mr. Skinny.

"Huh?"

"Your little voice is going through a growth process. We are trying to educate it and give it a stronger voice. I mean, make it louder and not just an afterthought. Your inner voice will serve as a guide to move you forward. And it seems like your voice is gradually getting louder," said Mr. Skinny.

"It is?"

"Yes! You're losing weight, not a lot, but you're losing and not from the workouts," explained Mr. Skinny. "It's from empowering your little voice."

Aubrey thought about how many times, while in decision-making mode, she heard a little voice telling her, "No," "I shouldn't," or "That's not right," yet she proceeded anyway. And each time she failed, that pesky little voice had been right.

"That little voice is your conscience. And what happens when your little voice contradicts what you want to do?"

Aubrey laughed and said, "I reason with it."

"Obviously, you outsmart it by finding a way to make your poor decision sound reasonable. You'll say, 'Oh, just this one time,' 'I've been good all week.' or 'You only live once.' Blah, blah, blah ... Sound familiar? Why do you sabotage yourself and let yourself fall victim to ... you? Be honest; close your eyes and think back. Your first inclination that ill-fated night was probably, 'No, I shouldn't do this.' Am I right?"

Aubrey silently laughed as she remembered that exact sentiment.

"And then somehow you talked yourself into it. Why do you do that? Focus on making a good choice now, this time, and as you move forward you will start to develop new habits. Each time you make a good choice; you will feel good and get closer to your goal. You can do this. I believe in you; I really do."

"Okay, I think I understand. My little voice is like my way of thinking," reasoned Aubrey.

"Well, kind of. What you are attempting to do is rewire your mental framework. Your relationship and association with food needs serious tweaking. Up until this point, every diet you have tried has failed," said Mr. Skinny as he put Aubrey on a treadmill.

"Not everything," said Aubrey, feeling attacked. "I have lost weight before."

"I don't count that," said Mr. Skinny, shaking his head.

"Why not?" Aubrey said, frowning her eyebrows.

"Because you gained the weight back; in essence, you never lost it."

"You see, Aubrey, it's like when your car breaks down. You become frustrated because you don't know what the problem is.

You look under the hood, move parts around, but aren't sure what is wrong. The only thing you know is that it must be fixed. You take your car to the mechanic and when it returns repaired, the world is right again. But then, next week rolls around, and BAM! It's broken again! You call the mechanic and say, 'Hey, it's still broken!' He counters back, 'No, I already fixed it.' You are infuriated because you know he never fixed the root problem. He solved a surface issue. The solution he provided was temporary; the underlying problem is still present. You need to get real and give me a chance to fix the real root problem."

Aubrey scribbled in her notebook.

"As we attempt to empower your mind and reshape your relationship with food, you need to remember that it will not be easy. Your mind will react in such a way that new choices will feel, well, difficult. But you will be prepared for these changes because you know they are coming.

"You see, Aubrey, it's like preparing to play chess. But in this case you know your opponent's next move. You know its strategies, how it will attack, and what methods it will employ. With this knowledge, you can formulate a winning strategy. You must create a winning strategy to win. There is no other choice. This is the process you are in now. You are training your little voice to handle situations in a new, powerful way; you are transforming from a passive pawn to a commanding king.

"The mind is fascinating. It acts like a preconditioned piece of machinery. You are, in actuality, a creature of habit. Your mind thinks and experiences life as it always has. In your brain, there are patterns of neurons called neural nets. These complex patterns of neural nets shape your way of thinking. This means that the manner in which you have experienced food and decision making is ingrained in your thoughts. Unfortunately for you, those old patterns don't align with your new goals. You must work to make new, better, more properly aligned decisions. As you form new decisions, new synapses will form in your brain. These new thoughts of fitness will form new thought patterns in your mind and will eventually feel good to you. But at the outset, it will feel different," explained Mr. Skinny.

"You see, Aubrey, it's like when you buy a new phone. You know that exciting, yet exasperating feeling when you start using the phone and everything is difficult? You think, 'How do I text?' 'Where's my calendar?' 'I can't see my emails' and 'I miss my old phone!'"

"Yeah, I hate that," replied Aubrey, wiping the sweat off her forehead.

"This period of adaptation is challenging. But then what happens?" asked Mr. Skinny.

"After a while, you learn how to use it, and in most cases the new phone is better," said Aubrey.

"My point is that in the beginning, everything will 'feel' hard. The choices will not be simple and these new thoughts will weigh on your mind. It might seem overwhelming. Please be patient as you traverse through the adaptation phase. This only occurs at the outset and it will pass. Remember the actual process. Your mind is trying to form new neural nets; these new synapses will work to reshape your way of thinking. And it will feel uncomfortable because it is a new thought process."

Aubrey was fascinated by Mr. Skinny's approach. He was taking fitness to a deeper level of understanding. She had never even attempted to get this level. Although the concepts were challenging, she felt she understood the main parts.

"I know it's a difficult concept, and don't worry about neural nets and the like. That's just for me to sound scientific and fancy," he smirked. "Do you remember watching rain as a child?"

"Yes," answered Aubrey. The question surprised her. She had no idea where he was going.

Window analogy

"You see, Aubrey, it's like that beautiful first rain of the year. As the fresh rain trickles down the window, it struggles to find a path. You watch the rain prance around looking for a perfect path to slide down. And then it finds that tract and all the other rain drops trickle down the same tract. The rain created a new tract; and if you watch this tract, it looks like it was there the whole time. This is how your mind is thinking and, more importantly, how your brain is functioning. With proper practice and the right habits, all these new decisions will become engrained in you. In fact, when you become proficient at this, you will wonder how you ever thought any other way. Fresh thought patterns will create a breathtaking new reality. But the only way to achieve this is through daily implementation of these new decisions. It is through habitual thoughts and proper decision making that you will see the dramatic effect associated with deliberate, positive actions."

Aubrey smiled and said, "Wow! This is compelling information. Learning the logic helps me understand what I'm doing and makes me surer of success!"

"You can do this, I know you can. You will excel because you are learning how the mind functions. Understanding the mind is fundamental to any successful fitness program," explained Mr. Skinny.

"Thank you so much, Mr. Skinny," replied Aubrey. "This feels different, unlike any other fitness program I have ever tried."

"You are correct, Aubrey. This is a completely different approach. Reshaping how you think about health and fitness is the key. I know that the way you think and what you comprehend will provide you the tools needed to last a lifetime. You are more likely to do something if you understand why. Now, for your third and final pillar, I want you to visit my friend, Drill Sergeant Dan," said Mr. Skinny.

"Are you going to enlist me in the Army?" said Aubrey as she chuckled.

"No, silly. Not the Army ... The Navy Seals."

Drill Sergeant Dan

Aubrey's jaw dropped, "Are you kidding?"

"Nope. You are going to attend one day of private training. There you will learn the solution to discipline. The drill sergeant is a master of discipline, which is essential to your success."

"I don't know if I can handle it."

"The physical part you can handle. The mental part, we'll see," teased Mr. Skinny. "I signed you up for Saturday morning's boot camp and asked him to spend some quality time with you."

"Gee, thanks," replied Aubrey. She was nervous about attending a boot camp and meeting a certified drill sergeant. *What will he think of me? I'm still pretty fat. He'll probably laugh at me. I hope Mr. Skinny knows what he's doing.*

The class was scheduled for Saturday at five in the morning, located at an actual Navy Seal facility. Aubrey was relieved when she learned she was not partaking in the physical activities. She was there to observe the soldiers training to become Navy Seals. At five a.m. on the dot, the soldiers marched out and began their exercise routine. The perfection, the cadence, and the sharpness of their movements was inspiring, a sight to see. Aubrey watched in awe as every soldier performed every task at the precise moment. The class displayed an incredible amount of accuracy and discipline. Even as the drill sergeant yelled, the soldiers held form and continued with their tasks. She watched them conquer an obstacle course. All the soldiers were in remarkable shape and showed no fear, even as they plunged into an icy lake. The drill sergeant continued yelling into the soldiers' ears. At exactly eight a.m., the class ended and the drill sergeant marched over to Aubrey.

"Aubrey?" shouted the drill sergeant.

"That's me," she replied.

"That's me, sir," he corrected.

"That's me, sir, sorry ... sir," said Aubrey as she wiped spit from her face.

"My name is Drill Sergeant Dan. I understand you are a friend of Mr. Skinny and need help with discipline." The sergeant spoke in a direct, loud voice.

"Umm, yes, sir," Aubrey said. She was embarrassed.

"Congratulations, ma'am. You should be proud of taking on this challenge," said Drill Sergeant Dan. "That takes courage and you need courage to have great discipline. What did you think about the class?"

"It looked great; the soldiers are well trained and disciplined," replied Aubrey.

"The soldiers are well trained and disciplined, sir," corrected Sergeant Dan.

"Oh, yes. The soldiers are well trained and disciplined, sir."

"Why do you think the soldiers are well trained?" asked the drill sergeant. "Do you think they come to us already disciplined and we merely put them together, or do you think discipline is learned?"

"I am not sure, sir."

"The final piece of the puzzle lies in that answer. You see, I know that you have a BIGGER BURN, a powerful desire to be successful."

Aubrey agreed.

"Those men over there, they possess a burning desire to join the most elite of all forces—the Navy Seals. That has long been their dream and their passion, and here is their chance. We only select the best, but each soldier must possess incredible discipline, dedication, and a strong inner voice. Their aspiration for success must ensure that they are brave enough to tackle the most dangerous of situations," continued Drill Sergeant Dan. "Any error, a second too early or a second too late, is failure; failure here is a matter of life and death. Unfortunately for you, your health is also a matter of life and death. You are borderline obese and it's time for you to get with it," said Drill Sergeant Dan.

Aubrey was alarmed by his bluntness. No one had ever called her obese to her face, and it hurt to hear from a complete stranger. But he presented his assessment as fact, without any emotion or judgment attached. Aubrey sadly knew the sergeant was correct in his analysis.

"You must realize, Aubrey, that discipline is the key to life's riches. It serves to separate the haves from the have-nots. When you are able to master discipline, and teach your inner voice the gift of discipline, you will see not only see your health improve, but your whole world will also improve," said Sergeant Dan. "Brian Tracy put it best when he described discipline as 'the ability to do what you have to do whether you feel like it or not.' That pretty much sums it up. Can you do what is required of you, even when you are not in the mood for it?"

Aubrey paused and said, "Yes, sir?"

"You don't sound confident. Why is this so difficult? Why are going to the gym, getting up early, and staying on task so difficult?" demanded the sergeant.

"Well, I'm lazy, sir?" she said as she straightened up.

"Yes! Plain and simple. Can you believe that? I offer you the world and you reply, 'I'm lazy.' You want to choose the path of least resistance; you want the easy route. Or my favorite line, 'I don't feel like it.' Really? That's interesting because I have never felt like paying my rent or paying for gas! I do it, not because I want to, but because I enjoy the benefits of a home and transportation. I understand that these are necessities for me to function," Sergeant Dan said, his voice escalating. "For your particular case, you must decide to eat healthy and participate in regular exercise. Doing so ensures that you will lose the proper amount of weight and increase both your emotional and physical well being. The benefits outweigh any perceived consequences. So, I am not going to ask, 'Hey, do you feel like doing cardio today?' I could care less if you feel like doing cardio. The question is, 'Did you or didn't you?' That's it. All I care about is the output. Did it get done?"

Aubrey felt scolded; she thought back to the numerous times she hadn't stuck to her plan by skipping the gym for her couch.

"Aubrey, you are at the tipping point. You need to make a change, you want to make a change, so let's make that change," shouted the Sergeant.

"Yes, sir! Yes, sir!" replied Aubrey. Everything seemed simple. Why was she giving herself choices? When given the choice between the gym and the couch, the couch always won. When choosing desert vs. no desert, desert it was. She clearly couldn't handle them? At least not yet. The message was clear, you don't get a choice, just get it done. Once her little voice was grown and well trained, she would be a well-oiled, decision-making machine. She started imagining it.

"Now, this is difficult to apply when it comes to food. How can you maintain the required discipline, day in and day out? When the motivation waivers, how can you stay on task?" asked Sergeant Dan.

"You're telling me … I mean you're telling me, sir!"

"Well, Aubrey, that answer will reveal the secret to success. I have not met one person who doesn't want to succeed. Everybody wants to be fit and be at their goals, but when we must make good choices, the situation is different. You need to pay special attention to that little voice in your head. That little voice that tells you what you should do and, more importantly, what you shouldn't do. This voice is skilled at revealing proper emotions when you do well and when you screw up. Correct?" the Drill Sergeant stared at Aubrey.

"Yes, I've had that ugly feeling of guilt, sir," Aubrey said.

"We're all guilty, Aubrey. I am not perfect when it comes to discipline. But I'll tell you the truth—I am better now than I was last year, and much better than five years ago. I have a strong inner voice that coaches me and helps me remember the pain associated with incorrect choices. That feeling: guilt. I don't like it; it makes me feel as if I did something wrong. And you know why?" asked the Sergeant as he lay his hand on her shoulder.

"Why, sir?"

"Because, I did! That's exactly the right feeling. And I hate how that feels, so I don't do that. I let the guilty feelings point me; if it feels wrong, I stop and change action. The reason it feels wrong is because it is. The actions don't align."

The sergeant stared into Aubrey's eyes. "If you truly want to make a positive change, accomplish more, and finally succeed, follow your heart and stay disciplined. When your actions align with your dreams, perfect harmony is attained and you are closer to complete empowerment."

"I need to empower my inner voice to help make the proper choices, sir," said Aubrey.

"Exactly. And when you make good choices for yourself, they are going to feel good. And when you feel good, you should feel proud."

Aubrey agreed; she was beginning to understand the power of discipline.

"It's okay to be selfish, Aubrey," said the Sergeant.

"I'm sorry, sir. What do you mean?" She scratched her head.

"We tend to think about selfishness in a negative light. Like it is forcing us to do things that we shouldn't be doing. But honestly, being selfish is okay."

She scratched her head again.

"Let me explain. Oftentimes when I begin to discuss the changes associated with proper food choices, people are quick to state, 'I don't want to deprive myself,' or 'That's no way to live.' Why do we feel like something is being taken away from us? It is this selfish attitude that has caused us to think that not having certain foods for a fixed amount of time will cause us an immeasurable amount of heartache. We act like the world is ending and everyone is against us.

"We need to stop that. No one is against you, and the fact that you are here in front of me means that you are ready to make a change. You are ready to be selfish, but in a positive way. You see, Aubrey, up until this point, you have viewed not having certain foods or having to set limits on food consumption as an external barrier that keeps you from fulfillment. The reality is that you can use those exact selfish thoughts to help you succeed. Be selfish, but not for food; be selfish for you and your self worth. Be selfish in knowing that you deserve to look and feel your best. Be selfish by treating your body like a temple. Be selfish by loving and respecting your body. Be selfish when others tempt you away from your goals. If you don't care about you, no one else will. No one, and I mean no one, cares about you as much as you do."

This struck a nerve deep inside Aubrey. She flashed through the moments when she was tempted her away from her goals. She remembered feeling deprived of her favorite foods. Those feelings were too familiar. She began to see the light.

"I guess I never really thought about it like that, sir," Aubrey said. "It's true; no one on earth will ever care as much about me as me. I need to take care of me for me."

Sergeant Dan nodded in agreement and said, "This is an important time, Aubrey, and as you prepare to make these changes in your life, you may start to miss the days of overeating. But remember, you've had your time to play.

"You see, Aubrey, it's like the dreaded summer school days. Remember the bad kids that played, skipped class, and didn't do their homework? Not a care in the world. And then what happened? Yup, the good times ended and off to summer school they went. Boy, was that painful; when everyone cheered fun-filled freedom, they were forced to attend school. Now stop and take a look at your life. Is it much different? You have enjoyed way too much fun. You have played and played; but now your play days must come to an end. It is time to face the music and place health at the top of your priority list. Up to this point, you have eaten whatever you've wanted. I'm sorry to tell you, but you overdid it. You really did. The sole reason people gain weight is from eating too many calories. If you take in more calories than you can physically burn, then you gain weight. There is no other reason. So don't fool yourself or lie to yourself. Accept it and move on."

Aubrey paused and took a few deep breaths.

"I know the truth is hard to swallow and you want to go to the doctor and have him tell you it's a thyroid issue or stress. You want something or someone to blame; that's easier than blaming yourself. But as I watch clients fail, I see the same pattern. When you have the discipline to accept responsibility for your actions, you are free to succeed," Sergeant Dan said.

"Your relationship with food is in desperate need of a paradigm shift. You need to focus on changing the way you experience food. I understand that food tastes good and it can enhance your mood. When you use food in this fashion, your dynamic with it changes. It is no longer fuel for your body. It becomes your source of instant gratification. It becomes a quick fix. You lose your ability to deal with your emotions and the result is that food becomes an external stimulant to cope with your feelings. But that is what you have done in the past; that is not what you are going to do from now on."

Aubrey nodded and left the camp feeling empowered. The MAD PLAN made more and more sense. Her fitness knowledge had improved and she realized why she had no chance of succeeding in her previous attempts. She made a promise to herself: her little voice would grow and she would do what was right, regardless of how she felt. The power of discipline would guide her through whatever challenges the world might bring.

The MAD PLAN

↳ *Motivation* ↳ *Accountability* ↳ *Discipline*

As Aubrey trotted to her workout session, she saw Mr. Skinny standing tall at the front of the Total Body Project gym. He had a smile on his face and said, "Aubrey, you are now ready!"

"I sure am!"

Aubrey had completed the foundation of Mr. Skinny's plan. The MAD pillars had been taught and implementation was next.

"Armed with motivation, accountability, and discipline, you are ready to take on your goal and ensure success," said Mr. Skinny as he handed her dumbbells.

"I really am, Mr. Skinny," said Aubrey. "I can honestly say that I have never been this prepared, motivated, or aware as I am today."

"Four, five, six, and rest ... and that, my dear, is the difference," replied Mr. Skinny. "Other times before, you may have had a plan with some unrealistic expectations. But this time, this time things are different. When you were trying 'Ripped in 90 days', 'Lose ten pounds in ten minutes,' or any other extreme program, you failed. Why?"

"Because I couldn't stick to it," Aubrey said.

"Of course you couldn't. You never had a chance because those programs don't work. Those diets are so restrictive and extreme that you cannot live the rest of your life like that. So, as soon as you're 'done' and return to your original eating patterns, guess what? The weight comes back! And let me ask you, Aubrey, when are you going to want to be fit?"

Aubrey's eyes lit up and she said, "Tomorrow, this summer, next summer, my birthday, my next birthday, actually my next anytime!"

"Exactly. All the time! I know we live in the world of 'now' and 'I want this today.' But trust me when I tell you, that doesn't work. If for some miracle, it actually does, those people become folk heroes. You've heard of them ... 'Well, my cousin did it and lost twenty pounds in three weeks!' Those people are the exception; that's why you hear about them. It's just like, 'My friend's friend invested in this penny stock and it took off and now he's filthy rich!' Eerily similar, right? What you are fighting here is basic human emotion. Human emotion places a higher value on the 'now.' Now is worth so much more! But what you fail to realize is that now will also be in the future. Our life is full of nows."

Aubrey raised her eyebrows.

"What I mean, Aubrey, is that the next now is coming. We always have now, but we have to work hard today to ensure that tomorrow's now is worth it."

"Let me see if I understand," said Aubrey with a faint smile. "My now today will also be my now in three months?"

"Exactly," Mr. Skinny said, smiling and winking. "Come on, three more ... Up to this point, I've had you log your food, write down analogies, and meet three powerful individuals. Now it's time to get serious and begin to move the needle. You see, knowledge is not power. Applied knowledge is power."

Aubrey placed the dumbbells down and exclaimed, "It's game time!"

"So, where do you see yourself? Exactly how much weight do you want to lose?" asked Mr. Skinny.

"As much as possible, as fast as possible," replied Aubrey.

"Wrong," said Mr. Skinny. "No, you don't." They walked past the gym mirrors.

"What do you mean 'no?' Yes I do," interjected Aubrey. "Look at my thighs, I hate them. I want them to stop making out! And I want it ASAP!" She shouted at her image.

"You say that, but you don't mean that. Let me tell you why. The ugly truth is that if you lose the weight too fast, your skin has no chance of catching up to the rapid changes in your body. That means that you will have extra skin sagging on your body. This is a sad truth that so-called weight loss experts never discuss. If you lose weight too fast, you will have issues with skin elasticity. That becomes a new problem to worry about," said Mr. Skinny.

"Oh no, I never thought about that," Aubrey was taken aback. "Gross! I don't want excess skin hanging off my body. Can I lose the weight without worrying about that?"

"Yes, of course. What you need to do is identify a specific goal with a certain time frame involved. I'll have you start with small goals and work from there. To accomplish your ultimate goal, you need to earn several wins. Multiple small wins will lead you to your greatest victory. In order to lose twenty, fifty, or even a hundred pounds, you still need to lose ten. And it's easier to lose ten than fifty. It is the same amount of work required to lose ten pounds as fifty pounds. The difference is the amount of time required. Let's start with ten pounds and give you five to seven weeks to accomplish it. Professional recommendations are about one to two pounds per week. As you learn these new skills, complete comprehension and understanding is most important. This will ensure your weight loss is not a fluke. You will learn and master these core principles. From there you can build. I promise you, if you stick to the plan, you will accomplish any weight loss goal, ten pounds at a time."

"Okay, I understand. Now, it's time to get me skinny!" Aubrey cheered.

Mr. Skinny smiled and said, "Ha ha, yes, yes it is. You are ready for the next stage." They walked to the juice bar.

"You have done well with your food log, writing it down helps, and for the most part, your food choices look more mindful," Mr. Skinny paused and looked at Aubrey. "Well, except for the weekends ..."

Aubrey shamefully smiled, "I know, my weekends are crazy, but I'm really trying."

"Yes, and it shows," said Mr. Skinny.

"Let me teach you more about calories and how they relate to your fitness goals. The first principle we need to grasp is the intrinsic value of calories, the 'what is what,'" said Mr. Skinny tossing and catching an apple.

Aubrey rolled her eyes and said, "I hate counting calories."

"I know ... I've heard that about a thousand times! What you need to understand is that you are not counting calories. You need to understand the value of calories; that is different."

"Go ahead," said Aubrey, "I'm listening."

"You see, Aubrey, it's like looking around the room and understanding the value of the items. Now you are not a pen or TV salesman, but you have some idea how much you should pay for those items. A pen maybe ten cents, a TV maybe a couple of hundred bucks. You need to also understand around how many calories food is worth. You need the ability to look at a plate, glance at a dinner table, and possess knowledge of the food's caloric value. If you have no idea, you have no chance. You will fail."

"Hmm," Aubrey said.

"Now, you won't get it right away, and that's okay. The important part is that you start applying 'what is what.' Use the web and search for food items. I also advise you to download a calorie app and start there. Begin inputting your food to find out 'what is what.' This will only be done in the beginning as you learn the caloric value of different foods. Eventually you will stop because you will gain an understanding and even begin to taste the calories," explained Mr. Skinny.

"So, I don't have to count calories forever?" Aubrey said.

"No, not forever; that is no way to live. Just until you understand what everything is worth, 'what is what.' A typical diet consists of roughly twenty-five to thirty-five different choices. As soon as you get the main staples down, you stop. Plus with your smart phone, when you are presented with a different food choice, you can whip out your phone and find the caloric value," continued Mr. Skinny.

"I think I understand," replied Aubrey. "I'm going to start learning the value of the calories and stick to a caloric budget?"

"Correct, Aubrey," said Mr. Skinny.

"Well, how many calories do I get?"

"Great question. The safe bet is to put a zero behind your weight and start there. For example, if I weigh one hundred and sixty pounds, I would start at sixteen hundred calories. But never eat less than twelve hundred calories," said Mr. Skinny.

They walked over to the scale and checked Aubrey's weight.

"I really hate this part," said Aubrey staring at the ceiling. She looked at the number and said, "Oh, my God. Wait, no, that can't be right!"

"It's okay, Aubrey. Today is a big day for you. Why? Because this is the first time you are not trying something short term, fast, and unsustainable. If you can accomplish these tasks and learn the underlying principles, you will be fit and happy for the rest of your life," said Mr. Skinny.

"Okay, so your caloric budget will be eighteen hundred calories per day," said Mr. Skinny as he adjusted the scale.

Aubrey said, "If I hit my calories, will I lose weight?"

"Yes, hitting your caloric budget is the secret to getting the results you desire," said Mr. Skinny. "There are other factors to understand too, namely the Caloric Conundrum," said Mr. Skinny.

"The what?" Aubrey's eyes opened wide.

"The Caloric Conundrum," said Mr. Skinny. "When we work with calories there are two problems. One, people overestimate the amount of calories they burn. Two, people underestimate the amount of calories they consume. Do you see the problem here?"

"Yes, the boundaries disappear," replied Aubrey.

"Exactly. What ends up happening is that when you think you are saving calories, you are subconsciously underestimating your caloric intake. This is challenging and you need to work to try and over report here. You will make errors reporting calories, but you want the errors to help, not hurt. Losing weight is difficult enough, but when you underestimate your calories, you think you're succeeding and then sadly this caloric mistake impedes your progress. Does this make sense?" asked Mr. Skinny.

"I think so. What you're saying is that the Caloric Conundrum tells us that when we report our calories, we tend to report less than we actually eat, or underreport? And that's bad, correct?" Aubrey scratched her eyebrow.

"Yes, when you underreport caloric intake, you feel like your weight should be flying off. In your mind, because you aren't eating as badly as you used to, you're winning. People will come to me and say, 'Well, before I used to have a large pizza and six beers, and now I only have half a pizza and four beers,' and 'I don't eat nearly as bad anymore,'" said Mr. Skinny.

Aubrey chuckled as she was guilty of that predicament many times.

"Just because you aren't eating as badly as before, doesn't mean that you are going to lose weight. You are eating better, and that's a good thing. But if your eating patterns were terrible and now they are just awful, do you really think that's enough to make a significant difference?" asked Mr. Skinny.

"Probably not," Aubrey shook her head.

"It feels like you are working harder, so you should be losing weight. But, in this case you are not looking at feelings, you are looking at facts. How much you consume versus how much you expend. Remember that although it feels harder, calories do not have feelings. They do not care whether you think you are working harder or not. All that matters is that you are in a caloric deficit. You need to eat a lot less and you need to move a lot more. When you move more than you eat, you are in a caloric deficit or a negative energy balance. Remember, calories are units of energy. Does that make sense?"

"Yes, I understand," said Aubrey nodding.

"There is some basic science involved, but you must understand the rules of the game to have any chance of winning," he said as he patted Aubrey's back.

"So, what should I eat?"

"You're asking about a meal plan?" Mr. Skinny pointed with his pencil.

"Yes."

"You don't get one," said Mr. Skinny, spinning his pencil.

"Huh? Why not? How am I supposed to know what to eat?" Aubrey placed her hands on her hips.

"Simple, Aubrey, meals plans don't work. When I go back to my days as a rookie trainer, I remember creating meal plans for my clients, tweaking them, and re-tweaking and re-tweaking, and you know what happened?" asked Mr. Skinny.

"They didn't stick to them," Aubrey looked down.

"You're right. It didn't work. Why not? Why would such a calculated meal plan that took into consideration protein, carbs, fats, sugar, and sodium not work?"

"It was probably too hard for the clients," Aubrey shamefully admitted.

Mr. Skinny placed his hand on Aubrey's shoulder, "I can't take people who are making major food mistakes and give them such a detailed program to follow. You have to learn to crawl before you can run. A lot of wasted effort goes into this. Excitement to create the perfect meal plan is intoxicating; people think they are going to do this and do that, and nothing gets done. Meal plans don't work. There is a small percentage of people that can execute a meal plan for a fixed amount of time, but they are few in number. Trust me, I have been in the fitness industry for a long time, and when fitness models and bodybuilders tell you what they are eating, they are lying. I am one of the most disciplined people on earth, and I cannot execute a meal plan, because it doesn't work."

"Okay, then what the heck am I supposed to eat?" Aubrey was agitated.

"Let's not be brash. Although meal plans don't work, meal planning works wonders. Let me explain. You already know what you should and shouldn't eat. Don't lie to yourself. Remember, there are between twenty-five and thirty-five different foods that you generally eat. You are going to keep those and work on lower calorie options. Everything that can be replaced for a lower calorie option needs to happen. You must try to find ways to shave off extra calories, because that's the name of the game," explained Mr. Skinny. "It's like cutting expenses for a budget. We need to find every single alternative that will cut even a few calories. But why would reducing only a few calories be important?"

"I don't know. Why?"

"Because you are looking for a marginal difference that theoretically will be sustained for the rest of your life. For example, if you save fifty calories switching from sugar to a sugar substitute. Well, that savings in your coffee happens every day. Let's do the math, that's fifty calories times seven days, which equals three hundred and fifty calories per week saved. Over fifty-two weeks in a year, you will save over eighteen thousand calories, or over five pounds per year. That's just the sugar in your coffee and only one year!" Mr. Skinny cheerfully pointed his pencil in the air.

"Wow! Five pounds from switching from sugar to a sugar

substitute? That's awesome!" Aubrey cheered.

"Look for incremental changes that can be sustained in your lifestyle. This will ensure that you are fit for the rest of your life. Analyze your current eating habits and find simple ways to gradually improve. My diet is clean, but this is after years and years of trying, learning, and growing. You don't start out by counting the grams in protein. That doesn't happen. Let's look at what you're already eating and find a way to make it fit in your caloric budget. And then you will work on it, day in and day out. Every day you will get better, every single day," continued Mr. Skinny. "Let's plan tomorrow's meals. Let's get a lunch box and pack your lunch. This will save you time, money, and most importantly calories. Remember as long as you hit your caloric budget, you will be successful. This I can promise you."

"But what about sodium and saturated fat and things like that? Do I need to worry about that?"

"Now, this is a point of contention. Many will argue that you should get something healthy, or organic, or gluten-free or whatever. But is this the real problem? Are we failing because our food isn't gluten-free or it has too many carbs? Is the color of the rice packing on the pounds? Stop making weight loss so complicated! It's obviously not the color of the rice that has gotten you to this point. It is the blatant over consumption of food and poor choices of high caloric food that has made you overweight. Making nutrition complicated will lead to failure. At the moment you have one concern, to hit your caloric budget. That's it. Whatever food choices you decide are fine as long as they fit in your budget. Hit your budget and you will win," said Mr. Skinny.

"Are you sure I shouldn't worry about sugars, or which berries have antioxidants?" Aubrey was troubled.

"Don't worry about that right now; that's all noise. For our purposes and for the position you are in now; it doesn't matter. Listen, one of the major pitfalls I see when people start on their path to getting skinny is they overcomplicate the process. In my experience, they are trying to sabotage themselves to make themselves believe they really tried. This is sad and confusing. But I hear it all the time. 'You see, I try to eat healthy and even diet soda is bad for me,' or 'I can't give up bread, I love bread.' Then the self-loathing talk begins. 'That's why I can't succeed; it's impossible.' They give up and go back to eating junk ... I get it. There is an inordinate amount of information on nutrition out there. And it's all great information that we don't need. I am talking about making choices with a deeper understanding. You are not there yet. You will get there, but today is not the day. Today I want you to stop eating so much chocolate cake. Let's focus on that. Let's take the confusing and make it simple. Let's simplify before we complicate. Let's do what works for you in your life and give you the best chance for success," he explained.

"Understood. When I can execute at this level, then I can move into a deeper level," Aubrey said.

"Exactly. Simplify before you complicate," said Mr. Skinny. "Your focus needs to remain razor sharp. Focus on the caloric intake and I promise you, this will work. But I do want you to worry about your water intake; it's better than when we started, but it still needs improvement." He pointed to her water bottle, which was full.

"I'm already drinking a lot. How much more do I need?"

"For water intake, I want you to take your body weight and divide it by two. Drink that number in ounces. So, you weigh one hundred and eighty pounds, therefore you need ninety ounces of water."

"That sounds like a lot," she sighed.

"It is. But the benefits to your health and weight loss are incredible. A good way to check is the color of your urine," said Mr. Skinny.

"The color?" she asked.

"Yes. If you have enough water in your system, it should be clear. If it's yellowish, bright yellow, or any other color, then 'Houston, we have a problem,'" said Mr. Skinny.

They both laughed.

"Sweet. More water, got it. So ... when do I start this new advanced nutrition program? Monday?" hoped Aubrey.

"Monday? Ha ha! Yeah right. You start now," Mr. Skinny said, pointing to his clipboard.

"Oh, now, as in today?" Aubrey threw her arms down.

"'I'll start on Monday' ... Why Monday? What's so special about Monday?" Mr. Skinny shook his head.

"I don't know, maybe the fact that I can get everything out of my system, once and for all," said Aubrey with a childish attitude.

"That's an excuse and more time to prolong the perceived pain associated with following a stricter diet," said Mr. Skinny.

Aubrey sighed, "I guess you're right."

"I know what you were thinking—one last hoorah, one last splurge, right?"

"Well," Aubrey shamefully smiled.

"Well, isn't it a fact that you have been 'hoorahing' this whole time?" Mr. Skinny tilted his head toward the mirror.

"I guess," Aubrey nodded.

"You see, Aubrey, it's like waiting until Monday to start saving money. Let's say you devised a master plan to save for your dream car by saving five dollars a day. You are excited about the savings to come. The daily sacrifice will lead you to realize one of your biggest dreams. Oh, what an exciting time! But the weekend leading up to your first day of savings, you spend three hundred dollars! Unfortunately, it will take you two and a half weeks to save what you spent. That sucks. I see this frequently with people. They sabotage themselves by completely overspending their caloric budget days before they start. They shoot themselves in the foot before the race starts! This isn't going to happen to you, right?"

"No, not me." Aubrey knew it was time to bite the bullet and get to the grunt work of the fitness program.

"Then commit yourself to change right now. Today is the best day to start your program. There is no prep work, no added mental preparation. You start today and you work until you get the body you desire. Come on, Aubrey, you have been waiting your whole life. You deserve the body you desire, and today is the day you travel a step closer," said Mr. Skinny as he bounced around.

Aubrey was mentally ready; she had been working with Mr. Skinny for a few weeks and her understanding of fitness had transformed. Where there was fog, the vision was now clear. *I truly understand what is important. I wish I would have known this before.*

"You know what? You're right. Today is the day, and the time is now. You have my full commitment to change," said Aubrey raising her fist.

"Congratulations, Aubrey. I am happy for you and I am sure that you will experience tremendous success. Now, go and grab your stuff. I am taking you grocery shopping," said Mr. Skinny.

"Really? Right now?"

"Yes, now. It's that important and the plan sounds simple; but failing to prepare for the week by not having groceries ready causes havoc on any nutritional plan. I am committed to your success; your success is my success. It defines me. I take pride in my profession. Honestly, Aubrey, the most important reason here is you," he smiled and gave her a hug.

Aubrey got teary eyed; she knew in her heart, Mr. Skinny wanted her to succeed. He was willing to do anything to help.

"I won't let you down," she replied.

"I know you won't, Aubrey. I know you won't," he said.

She changed her clothes and darted to meet Mr. Skinny, ready to go grocery shopping.

"This is fun," she said, beaming with excitement as she anticipated the new healthy foods that Mr. Skinny was sure to introduce.

As they walked to the grocery store, Mr. Skinny handed Aubrey a meal replacement bar.

"Here, eat this," he said.

She gave him a peculiar look and ate the bar.

"What is the bar for?" Aubrey asked.

"Well, a huge mistake that people often make is going to the grocery store hungry," he said. "You will make poor decisions and face too much temptation on an empty stomach."

That's true. Whenever I go to the grocery store hungry I end up getting food that I typically wouldn't.

"It's a classic miss, and it's easy to avoid with a little planning and some emergency food on hand," said Mr. Skinny.

"Emergency food? Wait, what's that?"

"Well, emergency foods are light snacks that you can store in your purse, car, office, or gym bag. These little snacks are there for emergency purposes, for the times you don't have access to healthy foods. For instance, if you have to attend a long meeting, a snack will help maintain your satiety and will prevent you from overeating later," said Mr. Skinny.

"Wow, what a great idea!" Aubrey said.

"Thanks, Aubrey, but I'm just giving you useful information. Remember, this will be your first successful time losing weight. Not only have I lost fifty pounds, but I have also helped hundreds of clients do the same. It's through years of experience, trial, and error that I give you the pertinent information. But it is still up to you to execute," said Mr. Skinny.

"Wait, hold on … you 'Mr. Skinny' … were overweight? Really?" Aubrey covered her mouth.

"I know it seems hard to believe, but I was once where you are," said Mr. Skinny. "I know what it's like to feel insecure. To avoid seeing friends because of the weight you have gained. To feel as if people are judging you when you go for seconds. To have everyone, and I mean everyone, give you diet advice."

Just then he reached in his pocket and pulled out his BIGGER BURN.

"Here I want to share this with you. A few years back I was

enjoying a nice Fourth of July barbeque. It was a typical summer day in sunny southern California. All was right in the world, or so I thought. We were hanging out poolside and there was another trainer there. Not a personal friend, but a cool character. He proceeded to take off his shirt, and this kid was in shape. He had abs for days and everyone stopped to admire his incredible physique. At this point, someone turned to me and said, 'Hey, Mr. Skinny, aren't you a personal trainer too? Let's see your abs.' I remember those words vividly, like daggers through my heart. Although I was in the fitness industry, troubles in my life had caused me to let myself go and I was nowhere near the kind of shape I should have been in. I felt embarrassed and ashamed. How could I ever help others if I couldn't help myself? At that moment, I made the decision to never feel that way again. It felt awful."

Aubrey stood mesmerized.

"It is for this reason, that if I am ever tempted to stray from my plan, from my goals, from my desires, I remember that moment and those awful, awful feelings. Never again. Never. I don't deserve to feel like that; no one does."

Aubrey nodded.

"I know the road is long and tough. But I also know how my life has improved. Nothing in life ever worth having comes easy. That's why I dedicate my life to empowering others."

They arrived at the grocery store. Mr. Skinny looked at Aubrey and asked, "Okay, we're here. Where's your list?"

"Huh, what do you mean? I thought you were going to help me buy all new healthy foods?" Aubrey looked around, confused.

He smiled, looked at her, and said, "Well, it doesn't work like that. First of all, why don't you have a list on your phone?"

"I don't know," she replied. "I just … kind of … try to remember what I'm missing and see how I feel," she knew this was a terrible answer.

"Without a plan there is no chance to succeed. Whenever you go to the grocery store, you must have your plan ready. Most people have a smart phone but don't employ all of its abilities. You should have a file on your phone that lists all of your food choices and whether you need that item. If it is not on your list, then don't buy it," said Mr. Skinny.

"What foods should I have on my list?" She asked as she took out her phone.

"Great question. What was the name of the game?"

"The Law of Conservation of Energy," answered Aubrey.

"Correct, and we want to minimize what?"

"Calories," answered Aubrey.

"Exactly," said Mr. Skinny. "Roughly how many different food items do we consume?"

"Between twenty-five and thirty-five," replied Aubrey.

"Perfect, so where should you start?" said Mr. Skinny.

"First, I need to work on getting lower calorie options for what I already consume," answered Aubrey.

"Bingo! Now, let's pull out your phone and start a list. This is the list you will use going forward. Remember, meal plans don't work, but meal planning works well."

They walked together through the grocery store and Mr. Skinny explained the caloric savings for each item they selected: diet soda for regular soda, sugar substitutes for sugar, cooking spray for cooking oil, popsicles, and the like.

"Now, the lower calorie options will taste different in the beginning," said Mr. Skinny.

"So what do I do?"

"You suck it up. Remember your BIGGER BURN and realize the importance of these choices. It's amazing to think that these simple items in your grocery cart will lead you to the body you've always dreamed of. I promise you, Aubrey, this will work," he explained. "Let's find enjoyable foods that fit in your caloric budget. You also need to find low calorie snacks, like fruits, vegetables, cheese sticks, or meal-replacement bars. You need to find items that you can munch on throughout the day to avoid long periods between meals."

"Do you know why that is important?" Mr. Skinny tossed oranges in Aubrey's cart.

"To keep my metabolism going?"

"That's kind of true. You need to eat every three to four hours to have a consistent energy level and avoid the starving feeling. If you go too long between meals, you risk overeating. You must actively work to avoid this feeling," explained Mr. Skinny. "Do you have a lunch box or a fridge at work?"

"Yes, I actually have a mini fridge in my office," Aubrey nodded.

"That'll work great, but I also want you to pick up a lunch box for those days that you are away from the office. From today on, you will always be prepared. You will not be surprised by life and the food dilemmas it brings," said Mr. Skinny.

As they finalized her shopping, Mr. Skinny stood in front of the candy and cookie aisles.

"Do you know what's in this aisle, Aubrey?" he asked.

She put her head down and admitted, "Yes."

"Okay, don't come down this aisle … ever. Why?"

"Because of the temptation?" she replied.

"Yes, that's true, but also remember why I am here with you. You want positive change in your life; you want to lose the unwanted weight. You want to be healthy. So when you or anyone else tells me, 'But, I don't know what I should eat,' I tell them to stop lying. You know exactly what to eat. But that's not what's going to hurt you. What is going to hurt you is eating the stuff that you know you shouldn't eat. You know what junk food is. It's crap. If you are serious about making a commitment to be healthier, why on earth would you put known junk food inside your body? Think about it … No, really think about it. It's called junk food! What do you think is going to happen? Stop playing games and start getting real. Sorry. I'm getting all fired up," said Mr. Skinny, shaking.

Wow, this guy really hates junk food.

"Aubrey, I know you have heard a lot about diets. All different sorts," he said.

"I know, diets don't work," she interrupted.

"Actually, you couldn't be more wrong. All diets work. They all work because they are all based on the Law of Conservation of Energy. All of them will put you in a caloric deficit," he told her.

Aubrey was confused. "No, you're kidding. I've tried every diet and they all failed," Aubrey said.

"The diets didn't fail Aubrey," he said somberly.

"What do you mean? If it wasn't the diet, then ... it ... must ... be ... Oh ... I see. The diets didn't fail, I did," she said.

"Yeah, diets aren't the problem, people are. Diets don't ever fail, but people fail all the time. It's an execution problem," said Mr. Skinny, pushing the cart.

"I see. Wow, now I see," said Aubrey said, smacking her head.

At the checkout line, Mr. Skinny said, "And one last thing. For Pete's sake, don't grab a candy bar on your way out. Control your snap judgment! A candy bar is about three hundred calories and wipes out an hour of cardio, just like that!" He snatched a bar and squeezed it as hard as possible. "Oops, I think I killed it."

They both laughed as they walked toward Aubrey's car. It was a Thursday night and getting dark. Aubrey remembered that she had dinner plans the next night with her friends, but she knew that one of her Accountability Allies, her sister, Sarah, would be there.

"Thank you so much for your help, Mr. Skinny, and for taking me grocery shopping. I really appreciate it."

"My pleasure, Aubrey. I want success for you. Now remember, one of your focal points is to have a strategy for the weekend. This first weekend is important," explained Mr. Skinny.

"Why?"

"I always like to start new diets on a Friday because the weekends are the toughest to get through. Most diets fail on weekends. If you start on Friday, when your motivation is highest, you have a better chance of getting through the roughest part. If you can execute through the first weekend, by Friday of the next week, you will have already lost weight and have momentum heading into the second week," explained Mr.

Skinny.

"Since weekends are so difficult, I need to really focus to get through them?" asked Aubrey. *That makes sense. I always thought of weekends as my time to cheat. I've never really tried to remain disciplined over a weekend. This is going to be tough. My sister's engagement party is this weekend! Oh boy, here I go.*

"Don't worry, Aubrey, I am going to be on call all weekend for you," he comforted. "Whenever you need me, text me the situation and I will give you a winning strategy."

"Thank you," replied Aubrey.

"Remember, you have your MAD PLAN in play. You have your motivation, accountability, and discipline working for you. Now you have to prepare your little voice for action on nutrition and ta-da! You are there!"

"Yay, simple enough," replied Aubrey, knowing that this task would be anything but simple.

"Go home, get some rest, and begin tomorrow with your new, lower calorie breakfast. Breakfast is important. Since you haven't eaten the whole night before, your body needs calories when you wake up. Breakfast should be something simple and predictable. I have found there is little variance with breakfast. People tend not to eat too many different foods, but stick to roughly the same choice, day in and day out," said Mr. Skinny. "What are you planning to eat tomorrow morning?"

"Cereal, with bananas, toast, and orange juice. Will that work?"

"That's perfect. Let's begin cutting calories there. That's a good breakfast, but I want you to check the serving size on the cereal, check the calories on the bananas and the rest of the food."

"Tomorrow?" asked Aubrey.

"No, right now. How many calories will be in your breakfast? Remember, you get eighteen hundred calories for the whole day."

She pulled out her phone and checked the caloric content. "This can't be right."

"How many calories are in it?" he asked.

"According to this, my breakfast would be six hundred and fifty calories, but that seems like too many," questioned Aubrey.

"You're right. I would actually guess that it's more calories than that. Because it probably says for a cup of milk, and a cup of orange juice, not a glass or milk poured to the top," explained Mr. Skinny.

"Oh, wow, this is going to require some work," said Aubrey with her hand on her hip.

"Only in the beginning, Aubrey. Start cutting there, maybe no orange juice, half a banana, and only one slice of toast. You will feel hungry in the beginning, but as you continue to eat smaller portions, your stomach will adjust and become smaller, or what I like to say: return to its original and intended size," he said, winking.

"I got it. I know what to do for breakfast," said Aubrey nodding faster.

"Great, so tomorrow through Sunday, I want you to text me all the time and let me know how you are doing and what you are having trouble with. You need to get your little voice trained and get prepared to take action on nutrition. This will prove to be invaluable, and you will then be cured," said Mr. Skinny.

Aubrey and Mr. Skinny exchanged good-byes and Aubrey went home. She knew that the next day would be the first day of the rest of her life. She had waited years for the answers to come, and they were finally here, but there was one thing left to do.

Here We Go ... Day One ... (Again)

As the alarm sounded at six a.m., Aubrey awoke armed with newfound fire. This was the most ready she had ever felt. She studied her BIGGER BURN and reflected. *Today's my day. Today I take care of me.*

Aubrey woke up twenty minutes earlier than usual. She had a bad habit of hitting snooze five to seven times before getting up. But since she started working out, her sleeping patterns had improved. Aubrey ate what Mr. Skinny suggested for breakfast, and made her breakfast shrink to four hundred calories. She even replaced the orange juice with coffee.

'Bfast Success,' she texted Mr. Skinny.

'Congrats! How does it feel?'

'Good ☺'

'Congrats on your first correct decision of the day. You probably feel all good inside because that's how good decisions feel: GOOD. Bad decisions feel: BAD. Keep making good ones and continue to feel GOOD.'

Mr. Skinny's remarks were surprisingly simple. Yet, when he said them, he had a knack for making them sound profound.

Aubrey packed her lunch box. It contained her food allowance for the day and also emergency snacks to store in her office fridge. However, as she exited the doorway, she stopped. ***Do it for yourself Aubrey, you have to do this for you.*** Her little voice grabbed a hold of her; she snatched a trash bag and in a flash of brilliance threw away all the junk food in the entire house. Getting rid of the temptations was a smart way to ensure success. The road was difficult enough. Why make it more challenging? The moment she threw away the junk food, she felt liberated. A huge weight came off her shoulders. *Now, I'm ready!*

Aubrey continued through her typical Friday. She was high strung and feverishly worked on deadlines. She glanced at the clock and noticed three hours had passed. *It's time for my snack.*

She ate a small orange and texted Mr. Skinny.

'At a girl, keep it up!'

'Now, Aubrey, lunch is approaching. Be Ready! In the past, you may have looked forward to lunch. Might have been your only pleasure in your day. If this is the case: change jobs. But that's a topic for a different day ;) Lunch cannot be your escape from the world and your reward for doing your job. You don't get points for doing your regular job. That's your job. Stop looking at lunch like some type of reward. It's not; it's simply another meal. Whether you packed or didn't pack your lunch, find a meal that fits in your caloric budget.'

'I got this, I'm ready.'

As lunch approached, a mad scramble commenced in the office. The faint sound of, "Happy birthday to you, happy birthday to you," began to fill the air.

Oh, that's right! Today is Carl's birthday! Ahh!

She grabbed her phone.

'Help! Office birthday party, and cake!' Aubrey was a sucker for chocolate cake.

'Relax, you got this. Your first major hurdle. Okay, I want you to practice what I like to call the Do Not Rock the Boat Strategy.'

'Remember, as you start your new life, people around you have no idea how you are feeling and you can't expect them to. Up until this point you have always participated in the gluttony. You can't be mad at them for offering you cake when you have always gladly accepted the cake.'

'That's true. I always get mad at people when I start my diet because I think they are out to get me. How are they supposed to know that all of a sudden I am not eating cake? That isn't fair to them. What's the strategy?'

'First, do not announce your diet. You will ostracize yourself and have uncomfortable discussions. If anyone brings up eating healthy before a binge meal, the mood changes. The crowd feels self-conscious. There is a time and place for everything; this is not the time. Take the cake, put it down, and decide what you will do with it. No one cares if you eat the cake. They only care that you accept it. It's a social gesture. If it fits in your caloric budget and you want some then have it, but it has to fit. That means A small slice (notice the emphasis on A). OR you take a bite, put it down, and walk away.'

'Really?'

'Yup, that simple.'

Aubrey joined the party, smiled, took the cake, wished Carl a happy birthday, and put it down. As the party subsided, she abandoned the cake, and nobody noticed. *Wow, no way, that worked?* Aubrey remembered previous episodes where she announced her diet and the room erupted into chaos. How she didn't need to be on a diet, and she only lived once, and that's no way to live, and it's my birthday. Indeed a hot mess.

She laughed as she skipped back to her office.

'It worked, and worked surprisingly well,' she texted.

'☺ Of course it did! Social gatherings are about celebrating people; the food is only a part of it. It's an offering that's ingrained in our culture. Celebrate people, not food.'

She smiled as she reread the text: 'Celebrate people, not food.'

Aubrey made it through lunch and felt excellent. All she needed to do was power through the rest of the day and go home. As she winded down at work, she received another text from Mr. Skinny.

'Now you have the Friday night dinner coming up and another big decision. I know what you're thinking: You know I work hard all week and deserve to go out and enjoy my dinner.'

She smiled and texted, 'Ain't that the truth.'

'You do work hard. But you've already enjoyed your dinners in the past ... That's why you are now where you are— overweight.'

'You've been there and done that, Aubrey. And where did that lead you?'

'Nowhere ...'

'How did it feel?'

Aubrey paused.

'Insecure, unhappy, and disappointed.'

'Those aren't good feelings. The time for change is now. Now you make a difference. Now, you make better choices. Making good choices makes you feel GOOD, really good. You deserve to look and feel the way you've always dreamed. Until you achieve that, everything else is irrelevant. Be strong, be proud, and remember to be selfish (the other way). You deserve this. Do not talk yourself into bad decisions. We as humans have the incredible ability to rationalize any decision. The convenience of being reasonable allows us to justify a wrong decision. Be good to yourself and watch how this beautiful thing called fitness comes to fruition.'

How did he know that Friday night dinner would be an issue? He's right. I was considering rewarding myself. But I always reward myself, which is how I got the body I have now. And the feelings I have now. That needs to change. I will make good decisions tonight and bring myself closer in alignment with what I want to achieve in fitness and in life.

Success! Aubrey picked a sensible dinner that fit in her caloric budget and felt proud. She heard the little voice inside her head, but this time the voice sounded different. It spoke with added authority and sounded like Mr. Skinny. She closed her eyes and heard:

> **"You should feel proud of your amazing work today. Remember, in the beginning it feels like a lot work and effort because it is. You are learning new skills and new habits and reshaping how your mind views these interactions with food. It is not always comfortable, and sometimes you might feel deprived. But that's okay. It will get easier. If you can repeat tomorrow what you did today, you will achieve greatness in fitness! Isn't that amazing?! That's it. What you did today, those simple acts, will get you the body you've always dreamed of! You are going to be hot, really HOT!"**

'I did it!' she texted Mr. Skinny. 'And I think my little voice is learning and growing. Is this it? Is this the secret to weight loss?'

'Well, Aubrey, the real secret lies in the application. The road may be long, but it's not any more difficult. Being in shape means that for the past year or so, healthy food choices outweighed bad ones. If you take each day as they come and find a way to win, you will be in amazing shape. Everyone will want to know what you did. Trust me. Life is made up of days, hours, minutes, and most importantly, choices.'

Aubrey went to bed with a tremendous sense of accomplishment. The knowledge and insight she gained gave her confidence. She felt in control and for the first time in her life, she believed she was going to succeed.

Saturday. No, Wait ... SATURDAAAYYYY!!

'Good morning, Aubrey,' came the text over the phone.

She sleepily picked up the phone and texted back, ':/ Morning.'

'Welcome to Saturday ... Well, it's usually not spelled like that ... it's SATURDAAAYYYY!!'

Aubrey's mood lifted and she texted, 'Yeah, Saturday!!'

Why is he texting this early? she thought. *Sheesh.*

'I am texting you this early because I want you to be prepared for your first big Saturday.'

'Huh? What do you mean?'

'Most fitness plans come crashing down on weekends. People relax their guard; a cheat meal here, a cheat meal there. Before you know it, they have blown all the savings they sacrificed all week for! One reckless meal can balloon to well over five thousand calories! That's two days of eating in one sitting!'

'Wow, really? How does that even make sense? That doesn't seem fair.'

'I know it's not fair, Aubrey. But much like life, it isn't supposed to be.'

'You see, Aubrey, it's like saving money. Saving money takes a long time, and a great deal of effort, sacrifice, and restraint. In order to save a thousand dollars, it takes ample time. Depending on your situation, it may take weeks, months, or maybe years. But to spend a thousand, or thousands, in seconds? Mind-boggling!'

'Yeah, that's true. Savings takes a long time, while spending happens in seconds.'

'Don't get me wrong, I get it. Saturday is here; it's your time to relax, party, and celebrate. But I'll let you in on a little insight; there is a Saturday every week. So don't be surprised or overzealous when it comes. Keeping that in mind, what's the plan for the weekend?'

'Well, I have my sister's engagement party today and a brunch tomorrow morning. That's it for the weekend, but I guess I'll give it my best.'

'Listen, you get fifty-two weekends in a year. Fifty-two! I am asking for three perfect weekends in a row, just three! If you can stay in a caloric deficit, you will lose an outstanding amount of weight.'

He knew it took twenty-one days to form a habit. If Aubrey could stick to three perfect weekends, she would have close to twenty-seven days practicing her new skills. This ensured enough time to see a noticeable change in her weight and for her to feel it in her clothes. Once she saw the results, momentum would help her stick to the program.

'Can you please do this, Aubrey?'

'Okay ... You got it! ☺'

Three out of fifty-two weekends doesn't sound too bad.

'Okay, let's plan for your sister's engagement. Isn't she one of your Accountability Allies?'

'Yes.'

'Perfect, I have a strong hunch she will have healthy food ready for you. But just in case, let me give you another food strategy.'

'Okay.'

'This one may sound silly, but you will be shocked at how well it works.'

'If someone offers you unacceptable food, look them right in the eye, rub your belly, and say: No thanks, I'm stuffed. I call that the No, Thanks, I'm Stuffed Strategy.'

"What? No, way. That works?"

'It's incredible how well this works. For some reason, people respect you for overeating and leave you alone. I believe it's because they want you be satisfied with the event and this gesture validates it.'

'Interesting.'

'Remember, events are about celebrating people. Food is a part of our culture and a part of the celebration, but not the main part. The people are most important, the people. The main component to understand at this juncture is the thought process and preparation for these particular situations. What are you doing here, Aubrey?'

'Learning?'

'Yes, but learning what?'

'How to say: No?'

'Yes, but you're not entirely correct. Look at the bigger picture. What you are doing here is formulating a game plan, a strategy for success. Your health is important and you do not want to leave it to chance or emotion. Figure out your big events for the weekend and allocate for them in your meal plan. My point is you shouldn't be surprised by these events because you knew they were coming. That's why they're called events! Don't be lazy; do the research to find out what will be served. Will there be anything remotely healthy? Drinks? Nachos? Chocolate cake? You need to know what will be served to formulate a proper game plan.'

Aubrey had never thought about forming a strategy for her weekend diet. She would have a meal plan for the week, and even exercise, but her weekend always had the "we'll just see what happens" attitude. Unfortunately for her, she saw exactly what happened. Having a strategy for the weekend was a clever idea to implement.

After Aubrey got dressed, she ate her small breakfast, a snack a few hours later, and then a light lunch. She ran a few errands and began to get ready for her sister's engagement party.

As she arrived at the celebration, her sister welcomed her with a huge hug.

"Aubrey, I'm glad you could make it," she said. Her sister worried, after Aubrey's divorce, that Aubrey would avoid anything wedding related.

"Of course, Sarah, it's your engagement party. I wouldn't miss it for the world," answered Aubrey.

Sarah whispered in her ear, "And guess what? I got healthy options for you."

Aubrey smiled; Mr. Skinny was right. "Awe, thanks Sarah, your support means so much to me."

"I know you're serious, and I want to be your rock of support," said Sarah.

"Thank you, Sarah. Thank you," she said as she looked over

and saw a healthy tray of delicious appetizers. Aubrey managed to have a nice time at the party, celebrating her sister's engagement. There was dancing, laughing, and drinking. Suddenly a server handed Aubrey a drink and she froze.

"Thank you," she answered. She whipped out her phone and texted Mr. Skinny.

'Help! There's a drink in my hand! What do I do? What about alcohol?'

'Good question.'

'Well, should I drink it or do I have to say good-bye to booze?'

'Well, again, this is up to you. Remember, as long as it fits in your caloric budget, you will reach your goal.'

Really? I always thought I had to give up alcohol! That's more like it!

'If I replace the higher calorie sugar-filled drinks with lower calorie drinks, that'll work?'

'Sure, even light beer is an easy way to shed calories. But remember, the major problem with alcohol is that if you get intoxicated, you tend to make poor decisions. And I'm not talking about calling an ex. I'm talking about overeating and eating things that you wouldn't normally, if you were clear headed. When you're drunk, everything tastes good. So don't eat carelessly. I promise, you will regret this. Either go to sleep, drink water, or eat something light in calories. It's usually not the alcohol that gets people, it's the late night runs through munchie fast food nation. If you can navigate through without a major setback, you will be on your way to success.'

Aubrey laughed in her head and thought back to all the drunk dialing and late night munchie runs back in college.

'Okay, I see. I'm not planning to get drunk tonight, but I was planning on having a couple drinks.'

'That's perfect, as long as it fits in your caloric budget. You will be fine. Enjoy.'

Suddenly, Aubrey's nightmare approached, dressed in caramel chocolate. Her favorite cake made a special guest appearance. This was the time to panic. She reached for her phone, but stopped. *Aubrey, relax, you can do this*, said the voice in her head. *You know what the right decision is; don't play games. You have worked hard and you don't want to let Mr. Skinny, Sarah, Carrie, and most importantly you down. Not today; today you will remain disciplined.*

As the server handed Aubrey the cake, she looked him right in the eye, rubbed her belly, and said, "No thanks, I'm stuffed."

Everyone at Aubrey's table laughed and carried on.

Congratulations, Aubrey, I'm proud, the voice said.

As Aubrey drove home that night, images of her new revelation overflowed her mind. She had attended an event where there was a possibility for overeating, desserts, and alcohol and she had stuck to her guns. The voice in her head, the BIGGER BURN, her sister's accountability, and her discipline had given Aubrey the strength to not just grudgingly get through, but to actually enjoy it. This inspired her as her previous thoughts of getting in shape required unthinkable, life-altering behaviors, where she would be sequestered and never allowed to have fun again. But in this new reality, there was balance. She jumped into bed thinking, *One more day and I'll have my first perfect weekend.*

Good Ole Sunday Brunch

'Good morning!' read the early morning text from Mr. Skinny.

'Good morning!' replied Aubrey, eager to start the day.

'One more day. Are you ready?'

'Yup, I have the brunch this morning and then I'll see you for our workout. I already went online to see what they are serving and I think I'm prepared.'

'Oh you are? Tell me.'

'The first thing I am going to look at is my budget. How many calories am I willing to spend at this event? Do I want to spend eighty percent of them there? If so, then I have to spread out the remaining twenty percent for the rest of the day. Correct?'

'Yes, correct.'

'Okay, I am going to have a very light breakfast (less than one hundred and fifty calories) and a very light dinner (less than three hundred calories), so I can use the rest of my budget at the brunch. Therefore, I get to eat about thirteen hundred and fifty calories at the brunch.'

'Exactly, and why will this work?'

'This will work because I am dealing with an energy question. How many calories I take in versus how many I burn. What I am actually putting into my body doesn't really matter when it comes to weight loss.'

'100% correct, Aubrey. Excellent job!'

Aubrey proceeded with her Sunday, executing her plan to

perfection: very light breakfast, and then left to brunch. Before she entered the restaurant, she reached in her pocket and looked at her BIGGER BURN, this always centered her. Especially when she knew she would be surrounded by temptation. The power of her message always motivated her in such a way that the rest of the world didn't seem to matter. Aubrey even went one step forward and moved her BIGGER BURN from her pocket to the background on her phone. Every time she looked at her phone, she would be instantly reminded of what was truly important.

"Hi, Aubrey," welcomed Julie.

"Hi, Julie," Aubrey said. She gave Julie a hug and kiss. Julie was Aubrey's long time high school friend. Like Aubrey, Julie also battled weight issues and suffered from similar insecurities.

"I'm happy you could make it," Julie said.

"Thank you so much for the invite; I can't wait to catch up with the girls," she replied. "What are we eating?"

"We're having the champagne brunch."

"You mean the buffet?" said Aubrey.

"Yes," said Julie.

Aubrey took a deep breath and said, "Splendid."

Aubrey you can do this. Remember what Mr. Skinny said. All you have to do is monitor the calories that you take in. Be aware and make good decisions. There will be other brunches, but today is about you.

Aubrey ordered champagne, with no orange juice, and asked to see a menu. Although the buffet looked delicious, she could not trust herself to make proper food choices, at least not yet. She searched the items and picked a larger meal than normal. When the waiter brought her food she asked for a box and cut her meal in half. The half meal was large, but she remained within her caloric budget. Aubrey looked at her friends and then down at her plate. She experienced a flurry of emotions; everything from envy, to temptation, to isolation. *Relax Aubrey, take a deep breath, and remember gatherings are about people not food. Celebrate the people.* She spent the rest of the time chatting up the girls. She had a fabulous brunch, but one aspect stood out. After all the talk about boys and the upcoming summer, she noticed the amount of calories that the girls were eating. It was the first time she saw how many mimosas, how much butter on pancakes, and the sheer number of pastries consumed. It was clear why she had never made any progress in the past. These meals were well in the three to four thousand caloric range!

Move, Move, and Move Some More

"Hello, Aubrey. It's great to see you. You're looking skinnier already!" said Mr. Skinny.

"Hi, and thanks. Yeah, my clothes are fitting looser and I feel healthier. I am getting this business of weight loss down, but now I see where I was making the biggest mistakes," she said as she jumped on the treadmill.

"What do you mean?" Mr. Skinny asked as he turned up the speed.

"Well, this morning at brunch, I was watching the girls eat, and mind you I used to eat like that. It didn't look too bad. But when I added up the drinks, pastries, and second helpings, some girls easily had about three thousand calories!"

"Yes, a huge problem and a classic misconception lies in that observation. I hear people talk about a cheat day or a cheat meal. I understand that a treat once in a while makes sense. But the harsh reality is that when you are trying to cut back on calories, one mishap can cost you dearly. Your friends' caloric intake in one meal was three thousand calories, but I like to interpret it in hours of exercise," said Mr. Skinny.

"How many hours of exercise?"

"For that one meal, I would bet around five hours of exercise," explained Mr. Skinny.

Aubrey's eyes opened wide.

"Yup, five hours. The human body exercising burns about six to eleven calories per minute, depending on the individual's size and condition. But a safe bet would be about eight calories per minute. That one meal, which was devoured in minutes, will cost her five hours of exercise! That one meal wiped out five hours, or a week, or maybe even two weeks' worth of gym time!"

Aubrey's eyes opened wider.

"I know, the ratio is skewed and it's not fair. So what? I'm not talking about fairness; I'm telling you the truth. When fitness instructors say you've burned over a thousand calories in an hour, that simply isn't the case," scolded Mr. Skinny. "That cheat day, that mishap, really cost them. And that's just one mishap; imagine how many other mistakes took place during the week! It's sad because they've probably saved the whole week and boom, in a flash, fail." Mr. Skinny shook his head.

"It's like you save five dollars a day for a month, and then you spend it all in one day! It doesn't matter how long you save, it matters how much you save!" exclaimed Aubrey as she ran.

"Ha ha! Yes, your first analogy. You are learning fast, grasshopper," cheered Mr. Skinny. "You got through the weekend and are ready to get back to normal Mondays. Now the process is easier and you are building momentum. Tackling nutrition through the weekend is one of the toughest tasks to accomplish. The weekends are of full of pleasurable land mines. I find weekends are the perfect time to start incorporating an exercise program into your daily life."

"But, I am already working out."

"Yes, you are working out with me and that's part of it. But now you are going to create your own movement program," said Mr. Skinny.

"A movement program? Don't you mean exercise program?" she said.

"Movement program, Aubrey; exercise is a form of movement, but it is not the only form."

Aubrey thought back to her energy equation, "Energy in versus energy out; the energy out must be all the movement?"

"Think back to the exercise programs you tried in the past," said Mr. Skinny as he handed her a water bottle.

She took a drink, remembered the crazy workouts that promised results in ten days, and said, "Hmm, let's not!"

"The workout program doesn't have to be some crazy ninety-day, butt-blasting routine. That may be a great workout; it's action packed, ridiculous, insane, and not meant for you! How do you know that?"

Aubrey continued to run, but said nothing.

"Simple, try one," he said. They both chuckled. "And when you can't hang and think it is too hard, you will be correct in your analysis. Fitness doesn't have to be a complicated fixation with all kinds of precision and specific routines. It boils down to making better decisions. It involves forming a skill set for a healthier lifestyle. Learning to value health and moving it up to the top of your priorities. My goal is to help you realize that fitness is not a distant wish that you strive to achieve; it's a realistic possibility that is a result of new, healthier actions."

"Aubrey, a fit person is someone who has made a higher percentage of healthy decisions. That's it. There is no perceived harder work. It only seems harder because you haven't done it, haven't completely committed, or more likely haven't had the proper approach. My clients have been successful in accomplishing these tasks. They truly understand the major fitness pillars. It is through an understanding of these fitness macro principles that individuals excel. Now, this is all fancy talk; what you need to understand is that if you want to get in shape, you need to move more and eat less. Don't worry about anything else. Everything else is noise. I've heard it all: How do I get my abs shredded? Lose the muffin top? Lose the love handles? I promise all of that will come in due time. As you master fitness, you will be ready and willing to train harder," he explained.

"Much like we did for nutrition: simple before complex, easy before hard?" she said as she wiped the sweat of her forehead.

"Exactly. Let me give you one of my favorite examples from the gym. I see a man starting on a fitness program. He pulls out the exercise routine of a famous professional bodybuilder, key word in this is professional, and begins the routine. A pudgy lawyer who hasn't worked out since high school is attempting the same routine the professional is doing!! What do you think will happen?"

"Nothing good," she joked.

"I want the lawyer to succeed, but what he needs is a program designed for a pudgy lawyer who hasn't worked out in twenty years!" he yelled. "I understand he wants to get a fit body fast. He wants to get skinny ... Now!"

"Ha ha! Yesterday if possible," she said.

"Well, sadly, you cannot speed up time, and I promise, if you could, you wouldn't want that. What if I said you would be in shape in one year and you could achieve it by tomorrow? All you need to do is sacrifice the experiences you would have, the memories, and the fun. Also, you'd be a year older. Would you want that?" asked Mr. Skinny, shaking his head.

"Well, no. Not like that. I don't want to miss a year of my life," she said, shaking her head.

"Exactly. People want to speed up time, but only when it's convenient. Unfortunately, it doesn't work like that. Good things take time. You wouldn't want a doctor who became one over the weekend. Like all good things, this process takes time; but it is worth it. As you start your exercise program, you will begin with easy and simple. Do you like biking, swimming, or maybe dancing?"

"Dancing? I love Zumba! Can I do that?" she hoped.

"Of course you can. Start with whatever you like; it can be the gym, active-play video games, hiking, or any physical activity that you enjoy," he bounced.

"Really?"

"Yes! Really! Anything that involves movement will work; but let me tell you a major secret," he said. "Come close, I can't let anyone else hear this ..."

She crept in close and Mr. Skinny said, "The secret is ... You have to do it!!"

She laughed, knowing exactly what he was talking about.

"For your weekend workout, pick an activity that you like to do, schedule a time, and go get it done. Plan to do this task at least once more during the week. With exercise, you will start with less, and as the weeks proceed you will add more."

"Why?" asked Aubrey. "Wouldn't you want more? That way if you plan for five and miss one, then you can at least go four times?"

"Another classic rookie mistake, Aubrey. You want to be in shape next week, next month, next year, and ten years from now. You need to employ a plan that will work for you for the rest of your life; a simple template that can be built upon. This will ensure success; easy now, harder later, when you are ready. As you continue on your fitness path, and you have proven yourself, you will challenge yourself more, maybe a 5K, a marathon, or an ironman triathlon. All of this will happen as you progress and you get in better and better shape," championed Mr. Skinny.

"As you begin your fitness journey, I want you to place most of your energy on mastering that basic equation: Energy in versus energy out. Incorporate more movement in your day. How can you do this?" asked Mr. Skinny, tapping the pencil on his clipboard.

Aubrey thought for a moment. She has an office job which is sedentary and provides little movement. Then her inner voice came in strong: *Find a way, Aubrey. Don't accept why not. I want to hear in spite of this obstacle, I was able to ...*

"At your office," started Mr. Skinny.

"I can take the stairs and I can park farther away!" she cheered.

Mr. Skinny smiled and said, "I see your inner voice is taking command. And do you see how these changes in movement will help you?"

"More movement means I expend more energy, which means I burn more calories, right?" asked Aubrey as they looked up the gym stairs.

"That's correct. Let's look at the value of these new movements. On the surface it may not seem like much. So you take the stairs to the office. Big deal, right? Well, it kind of is. Let's do the math. If you're on the third floor and you take the stairs twice a day, you burn roughly twenty calories in those three minutes walking up, and that happens daily for five days, and for twelve months, so in a year that's twenty-four hundred calories. That may not seem like a lot now, but what about over the next twenty years? How many calories is that?" he asked at the top of the stairs.

"That's forty-eight thousand calories!" she clapped.

"Yes, or how many pounds? Remember divide calories by thirty-five hundred," he said.

"About ... fourteen pounds! Wow! And only from taking the stairs at work!"

"Now, if you park farther away ..."

Aubrey smiled and nodded.

"You get the picture, what we are looking for is incremental behavioral changes that you can sustain to increase the caloric expenditure over your lifetime. This will make a bigger difference in getting you skinny than any one-hour exercise program," he explained. "The name of the game is how can you burn more calories, increase your movement, burn more, increase movement," he said.

"That's simple. I like that," Aubrey said.

"Yes, these are simple behavioral changes that can be employed daily. The only reason why you wouldn't do them is because you are either lazy or don't know the importance of movement. If you do this, Aubrey, it's only a matter of time before you have the body of your dreams. But you can't be lazy anymore," he said.

"I promise I won't be lazy anymore," she said.

"Now that you have the knowledge, you must apply it. The choice is yours. The parade is coming, that's for sure. You can either be in the parade or you can watch the parade pass you by. What I am trying to tell you is that you can and will be successful with these proven tactics," said Mr. Skinny.

Aubrey felt more alive and ready than she had ever felt. She had confidence in her inner voice and knew her new fitness strategies would work. She sensed that her time with Mr. Skinny was coming to an end.

"How can I ever repay you?"

Mr. Skinny paused and said, "There are two promises that I ask of you."

"Of course, anything," Aubrey said.

"The first is to promise me that you will employ these fitness principles, reach your goals, and have the body you've always dreamed of. My goal is to empower you with confidence not only in your appearance but also in your attitude toward life. These fundamental fitness principles will show you the simplicity and true beauty of fitness. Your success is the ultimate way to repay me."

"You got it. I will make you proud, Mr. Skinny," championed Aubrey. "What's the other promise?"

"As you know, obesity is becoming an epidemic. It saddens me to watch people compromise their lives because of a lack of education. Many have the desire, but desire without the right plan leads nowhere. The fitness world can be confusing. Fitness has enhanced my life in countless ways; I believe it's a gift that everyone deserves to possess. Share these fitness principles with those you hold dearest and watch in amazement. As their lives improve, so will yours. Together we can all be fit and healthy, and lead fulfilling lives. Living life the way it was meant to be, absolutely amazing!"

Sweet, Sweet Success!!

"Good morning, Aubrey. Can I talk to you?" asked Carrie.

"Of course, come right in," replied Aubrey.

Carrie sighed and said, "I want to ask for your help."

"Sure, what can I help you with?"

"Well, I want to know your secret."

"My secret? My secret for what?" answered Aubrey.

"Your secret for how you have done it. In the last eight months, you have been on fire. You got promoted to executive, you have a new boyfriend that treats you amazingly, you completed your first half marathon, you work out, you are always going out and ... and ..."

Aubrey smiled and said, "... and?"

"You're so freaking skinny! Get me Skinny!!" shouted Carrie.

Aubrey smiled and said, "Awe, thanks Carrie, but you know as well as I do that the path wasn't easy."

"I know. And I know you worked with Mr. Skinny. But honestly, I can't afford him," Carrie said, shaking her head.

This saddened Aubrey. She, like Mr. Skinny, wanted everyone to have fitness success in their lives.

"I got it!" exclaimed Aubrey. She reached in her drawer and pulled out a beat-up notebook.

"Here, take this," said Aubrey.

Carrie opened the notebook and on the left side were Aubrey's meals from when she started with Mr. Skinny. On the right side were Mr. Skinny's Power Analogies, complete with the MAD PLAN.

Carrie opened the notebook:

M—Motivation   **P**—Prepare the

A—Accountability   **L**—Little Voice for

D—Discipline   **A**—Action on

N—Nutrition

BIGGER BURN

Find your ultimate "why."

Accountability Alliance

Choose 3 people to hold you accountable, one at work, one at home, and your closest friend.

Discipline

Do what you have to do, whether you feel like it or not.

1 pound = 3,500 calories

To lose a pound, you must burn 3,500 calories.

Law of Conservation of Energy

The only equation that matters.

ENERGY IN vs. ENERGY OUT

Calories In: *Food Intake* vs. Calories Out: *Activity Level*

Eat Too Much + Move Too Little = **Gain Weight** =>
Store Extra Calories (FAT) ☹

Eat Less + Move More = **Lose Weight** =>
Drop Excess Calories (LEAN) ☺

Proper Diet + Moderate Activity = **Maintain Healthy Weight** *(MAINTAIN)*

Nutrition: Add a Zero for Caloric Intake

To lose weight, add a zero to your weight, and that's your reduced caloric intake. As your weight goes down so will the calories. But no less than 1200 calories.

Ex. 180 lbs -> 1800 calories

Water: Divide Weight by 2 in Ounces

To lose weight, take your weight, divide by two and convert to ounces, and that's how much water you need.

Ex. 180 lbs -> 90 ounces

The Caloric Conundrum

1. *People overestimate the amount of calories they burn.*
2. *People underestimate the amount of calories they consume.*

Small Wins Lead to Great Victory

> Meal Planning vs. Meal Plans

What Is What

> Emergency Food

Simplify Before You Complicate

> Celebrate People, Not Food

Do Not Rock the Boat Strategy

> No Thanks, I'm Stuffed Strategy

One Bad Meal = Five Hours of Exercise

> Movement Program

Mr. Skinny's Power Analogies

#1

Your weight loss journey is like traveling through a strange forest. You don't know the exact way or how far or how treacherous the quest will be. The true perils of the forest lie in the unknown. How can you survive alone? I, on the other hand, have been through the forest many times. I have safely traversed the difficult paths with a variety of people, taking special note of each of their strengths and providing an appropriate course. Not only can I map the route, I also know the fastest, safest, and most secure way. So listen intently, follow closely, and enjoy the fruits of success.

Listen and follow the advice. I haven't done it before, but he has many times with many different people. He's the expert.

#2

Your fitness level is like a choice scale. You need to analyze all of your choices for the past year on this imaginary balance scale. On the left side you have all the year's bad choices, and on the right side you have all the good choices. In your particular case, you are skewed to the left. Your balance has more bad choices than good ones. As you begin to positively move forward, the scales will tilt in your favor. Slowly but surely, you will add more good choices and the balance will tilt toward the middle. When the scale is balanced, you will have just as many good choices as bad choices. But to make real progress, you need more good choices. You need to be good a lot longer than you were bad.

I look the way I look based on the decisions I have made over the past year. If I look poorly, it's because I've made poor decisions for my health. If I want to look better, I need to make better choices over the course of the next year.

#3

Taste interpretation is like Thanksgiving dinner. We know it as a day to not only feast, but to gorge. To let loose and eat anything and everything our little hearts desire. Most people wait the whole day, refusing to eat until dinner, and end up starving themselves. They starve themselves with one intention: when the special dinner arrives in their tummy, it will have the taste of legends. Now, let's take the same meal, spectacular and everything. What happens if you eat an apple right before? What happens to the legendary taste, the meal fit for kings? It doesn't taste the same, does it? It tastes ordinary. Does that strike you as odd? The actual food composition hasn't changed one bit. The difference is how our mind interprets the food. It's fascinating.

If I wait too long between meals, the way my mind interprets taste completely changes. Because I am in "starving" mode, I crave fattier foods. Craving fattier foods somehow makes them taste better. I need to avoid this craving because it leads to overeating.

#4

Managing calories is like managing money. If you want to lose weight, burn more calories than you eat. If you want to be rich, make more money than you spend. Pretty simple, huh? The difference is that with money you have precise vision. When you are the beneficiary of a raise or a gift, you know exact numbers. If you overspend money, you see your account balance drop. Unfortunately, this isn't the case with food. Without being able to see your food balance, you are forced to guess. You have to guess at how many calories you take in and how many calories you burn. Sadly, you usually guess in your own selfish favor.

To lose weight, I need to burn more calories than I eat. Not being able to see my caloric balance forces me to guess. This makes it harder to lose weight.

#5

Fitness accountability is like that ten-page paper that you had due in college. Remember those good old college days when you looked at the syllabus and thought, 'That's not due till week seven, I have plenty of time'? And there you found yourself, trying to print your paper minutes before it was due. But, you got it done. Why? Because it was being collected. You were being held accountable. For weight loss, this 'paper' you have to turn in gets collected when? Never. So what happens? You procrastinate and don't get it done. And if you make horrible nutrition choices, the 'paper' gets longer. You forget to work on it, and you get the point. Nothing happens. With no one there to check your progress, you can only hold yourself accountable, which might not be a good thing.

When there is no accountability for my weight loss goals, I won't finish them. If left to my own devices, I will procrastinate and never complete my goal.

#6

An Accountability Alliance is like the stick story. Let's say you are in the woods gathering sticks. One stick is easy to break; but if you pick up another similar stick and try to break them together, the sticks are more resilient. You pick up a third stick and even more strength is added. The sticks together are stronger than any stick individually.

By asking the people closest to me to help, they provide a higher level of accountability and, thus, my problem becomes our problem. In this manner, we work as a team to help me succeed.

#7

Setbacks are like trying to dig a hole. Picture a mountain of sand, which represents all the calories that you have overeaten throughout the years. For you to succeed, you need a hole in that mountain of sand. Better get to digging. You grab your small shovel and work diligently to dig a deep hole. Digging, digging, day in and day out, working laboriously, covered in sweat through fall, winter, and spring. You pause to take a break and leave your hole unattended. A dump truck zooms in and drops a load of sand into your hole! That momentary lapse in judgment cost you your countless hours of digging in a matter of seconds. Mistakes are setbacks and are part of life, but you must learn from them. You may want to give up, but you still need to dig. And dig a lot. You can't give up. You have no other choice.

It really doesn't matter how long I work on my goal. If I have a setback, the setback can cost me severely. The time spent dieting can all be eliminated with a single bad decision. Time has no relation to the amount of calories ingested.

#8

Permanent fitness success is like when your car breaks down. You become frustrated because you don't know what the problem is. You look under the hood, move parts around, but aren't sure what is wrong. The only thing you know is that it must be fixed. You take your car to the mechanic and when it returns repaired, the world is right again. But then, next week rolls around, and BAM! It's broken again! You call the mechanic and say, 'Hey, it's still broken!' He counters back, 'No, I already fixed it.' You are infuriated because you know he never fixed the root problem. He solved a surface issue. The solution he provided was temporary; the underlying problem is still present. You need to get real and give me a chance to fix the real root problem.

In the past when I lost weight and gained it back, I never really lost it to begin with because I never fixed the real problem. I never understood "how" to lose the weight. That doesn't count.

#9

Proper fitness mental programming is like preparing to play chess. But in this case you know your opponent's next move. You know its strategies, how it will attack, and what methods it will employ. With this knowledge, you can formulate a winning strategy. You must create a winning strategy to win. There is no other choice. This is the process you are in now. You are training your little voice to handle situations in a new, powerful way; you are transforming from a passive pawn to a commanding king.

I can prepare my mind for the obstacles that lay ahead. With this method, I can assure myself of success, with no surprises. I need to teach my mind to think properly when faced with tough challenges.

#10

Learning new skills is like when you buy a new phone. You know that exciting, yet exasperating feeling when you start using the phone and everything is difficult? You think, "How do I text?" "Where's my calendar?" "I can't see my emails," and "I miss my old phone!"

In the beginning, all actions seem difficult, but it is only the beginning. Soon, these new thoughts and skills will become easy and a part of me.

#11

New thought patterns are like that beautiful first rain of the year. As the fresh rain trickles down the window, it struggles to find a path. You watch the rain prance around looking for a perfect path to slide down. And then it finds that tract and all the other rain drops trickle down the same tract. The rain created a new tract; and if you watch this tract, it looks like it was there the whole time. This is how your mind is thinking and, more importantly, how your brain is functioning. With proper practice and the right habits, all these new decisions will become engrained in you. In fact, when you become proficient at this, you will wonder how you ever thought any other way. Fresh thought patterns will create a breathtaking new reality. But the only way to achieve this is through daily implementation of these new decisions. It is through habitual thoughts and proper decision making that you will see the dramatic effect associated with deliberate, positive actions.

The way I think today is the direct result of yesterday's thoughts. In order to form new habits, I have to practice new ways of thinking. These new ways of thinking will lead me to new and improved habits. The right habits will get me the body I have always wanted.

#12

Fitness discipline is like the dreaded summer school days. Remember the bad kids that played, skipped class, and didn't do their homework? Not a care in the world. And then what happened? Yup, the good times ended and off to summer school they went. Boy, was that painful; when everyone cheered fun-filled freedom, they were forced to attend school. Now stop and take a look at your life. Is it much different? You have enjoyed way too much fun. You have played and played; but now your play days must come to an end. It is time to face the music and place health at the top of your priority list. Up to this point, you have eaten whatever you've wanted. I'm sorry to tell you, but you overdid it. You really did. The sole reason people gain weight is from eating too many calories. If you take in more calories than you can physically burn, then you gain weight. There is no other reason. So don't fool yourself or lie to yourself. Accept it and move on.

I had my time to screw around. Now it's time to pay the piper and get to work.

#13

Intrinsic caloric value is like looking around the room and understanding the value of the items. Now you are not a pen or TV salesman, but you have some idea how much you should pay for those items. A pen maybe ten cents, a TV maybe a couple of hundred bucks. You need to also understand around how many calories food is worth. You need the ability to look at a plate, glance at a dinner table, and possess knowledge of the food's caloric value. If you have no idea, you have no chance. You will fail.

I don't need to count calories, but I must have an idea of how many calories foods possess. I need to have a clue to what is worth what, which will help me eliminate extraordinarily high caloric foods.

#14

Saving calories is like waiting until Monday to start saving money. Let's say you devised a master plan to save for your dream car by saving five dollars a day. You are excited about the savings to come. The daily sacrifice will lead you to realize one of your biggest dreams. Oh, what an exciting time! But the weekend leading up to your first day of savings, you spend three hundred dollars! Unfortunately, it will take you two and a half weeks to save what you spent. That sucks. I see this frequently with people. They sabotage themselves by completely overspending their caloric budget days before they start. They shoot themselves in the foot before the race even starts!

If I am serious about achieving my goal, don't give myself more work. It's already hard enough to lose weight, don't add more calories during the weekend only to start burning them off on Monday. Start now before any more damage is done.

#15

Burning calories is like saving money. Saving money takes a long time, and a great deal of effort, sacrifice, and restraint. In order to save a thousand dollars, it takes ample time. Depending on your situation, it may take weeks, months, or maybe years. But to spend a thousand, or thousands, in seconds? Mind-boggling!

Burning calories takes effort. Losing weight requires more effort. But eating calories and gaining weight is way easier. It's not fair, but that's just the way it is.

Carrie closed the notebook and with tears in her eyes said, "Aubrey, thank you for this. How can I ever repay you?"

Aubrey smiled and said, "Promise me that you will employ these fitness principles, reach your goals, and have the body you've always dreamed of. My goal is to empower you with confidence, not only in your appearance, but also in your attitude toward life. These fundamental fitness principles will show you the simplicity and true beauty of fitness. Your success is the ultimate way to repay me."

Carrie hugged Aubrey and said, "Thank you, thank you. Can I at least treat you to happy hour Friday night?"

"Happy hour?" Aubrey paused for a moment. She hadn't dared to attend happy hour in over eight months.

"Happy hour will be just ... perfect. There is a certain someone I hope to bump into again." A sly smile swept across Aubrey's face.

Appendix

Movement Program

1. Schedule regular exercise
2. Fidget
3. Take the stairs
4. Park farther away
5. Exercise while watching TV
6. If getting fast food, exit car
7. Join a recreation league
8. Incorporate circuit training
9. Clean your house
10. Stand to make calls
11. Move cell phone further away
12. Move printer further away
13. Walk during lunch
14. Put down the remote
15. Stand vs. sit
16. Sit vs. lie
17. Bike to work
18. Walk your dog
19. Play with the kids
20. Shop
21. Wash dishes by hand
22. Garden
23. Sex
24. Dance

Exercise to Food Ratios:

Beer + Beer + Beer + Chips = 2 hours, 25 mins of Running

Donut + Donut +Flavored Coffee = 1 hour, 25 mins of Swimming

Slice of Cake + Slice of Cake = 1 hour, 33 mins of Cycling

Cheeseburger + Fries + Soda = 3 hours of Basketball

Testimonials

"Tony was by my side for a year, shedding his own sweat, blood and tears as he helped me prepare for my wedding day. But the most important thing that I have gained from Tony's impact on my life is the confidence to go out and start really living my life. I felt phenomenal in my wedding dress, not because of the body Tony had helped me to achieve, but because of the confident person Tony had helped me become. It isn't just about losing weight or fitting into a wedding dress; it is about a lifestyle change. Tony makes it so simple with his philosophy. There are no complicated meal plans or weird shakes to drink every two hours, like other trainers I have had and diets I have tried."
-Nicole Collins Cannis, Audit Supervisor, MTC Financial

"Over the five month period I lost 18 pounds and improved my strength and cardio fitness to the best level of my life! I even improved my golf game! I am very grateful to Tony."
-Dr. Phillip Quirk, M.D.,Kaiser Permanente

"Not only is Tony knowledgeable about various aspects of fitness, he is also extremely attentive as a personal trainer and is 100 percent focused on me as a client-something that I should underscore is an important trait for any personal trainer...Finally, a world about Tony's interpersonal skills-he is bright, energetic, enthusiastic, and motivating."
-Dr. Jennifer Lee, Professor, UC Irvine

"Tony has not only demonstrated that he can get you results, but teaches you to continue eating healthy and exercising for life not just while training. You develop the strength and power to confidently care about your internal and external beauty."
-Nadia Gomez, Teacher, CA

"Training with Tony quickly became much more than just a diet and exercise plan. It became a place to relieve stress, continue to set new goals, and push my boundaries both physically and mentally. I don't consider myself to be a very athletic person and would have never thought to compete in any endurance events and here I am, 5 half marathons later, training for my first full marathon. This drive to continuously improve has transferred to other aspects of my life and I believe it has helped me greatly with my career and personal life as well."

-Jose Martinez, Engineer, Mazda Corp

"His work ethic, enthusiasm, passion, knowledge, professionalism, and the pure joy he gets from making you reach YOUR goals are simply among many commendable qualities Tony possesses. I have been with Tony for the past 8 months and my body was completely transformed 4 months in! The way I think of my goals and my mindset is also in a state of transformation, thanks to Tony."

-Laily Boutaleb, Esq. Army JAG Officer

"Exactly 6 months ago, I was a candy-addict that would love to eat junk food. I decided to change my lifestyle when I found out how unhealthy I was. I started at 222 pounds and 26% body fat. Today, after 6 months of hard work and sacrifices, I am NOW 176 pounds, and 15.1% body fat! I couldn't be more proud of myself! I want to thank the person that made all this possible, Tony Arreola. I don't know what I would do without him. Thank you."

-Fausto Villanueva, MBA Student, USC

About the Author

Tony Arreola

A certified personal trainer who enjoys every second of what he does, Tony Arreola has been immersed in the fitness industry for as long as he has lived. Tony entered UC Irvine with an engineering career on his mind. It was there that his passion for helping and teaching people truly flourished. He served as a tutor, mentor and teacher throughout his UCI career. Tony found his calling as he inspired his college roommate to lose fifty pounds. The fifty pounds that his roommate lost completely transformed both of their lives. One enjoyed a new physique, new found confidence, and true happiness; the other found his life's mission.

After college, he began a career as a personal trainer for 24 Hour Fitness. Tony thrived, becoming a stand out trainer, a fitness manager and eventually holding the title of general manager. After 24 Hour Fitness, Tony decided to take a leap of faith, and form Total Body Project. His dream: to bring fitness success to everyone who desires it.

Tony has helped hundreds of clients lose thousands of pounds, with an incredible 90% client success rate. But his true gift is his ability to explain fitness in simple, understandable terms. Tony has three certifications from the National Academy of Sports Medicine (NASM) and holds two degrees, one in Engineering and the other in Economics. He believes that education is the key to fitness and life empowerment.

Tony resides in Irvine, California where he lives his passion every day. He is an active triathlete whose life goal is to complete an Ironman triathlon, every year in a different part of the globe until he turns 100!

Stay Connected

Visit Our Website
Go to **www.totalbodyproject.com** to learn more about us and our services. Learn about new books, fitness videos, personal training services, gyms and fitness products.

Fitness Seminars
Want Mr. Skinny to present at your company? Mr. Skinny presents fun fitness presentations designed to keep the workforce happy, healthy and fit.
For Bookings: *tonyarreola@totalbodyproject.com*

Like our Total Body Project Page on Facebook
Join our fitness community. Hear more success stories from people like you. Get fitness tips and daily motivators.

Become Mr. Skinny's Friend
Stay motivated, stay positive and let Mr. Skinny help you on your real life fitness journey.
Add Tony Arreola on Facebook

Subscribe to Our Newsletter
Be the first to learn of new products, and exciting new ways to make the game of fitness, a simple winnable one.
Send a request to*: **tonyarreola@totalbodyproject.com***

Follow Mr. Skinny on Twitter
Receive timely thoughts and information on Mr. Skinny's daily events*: **tonyarreola@tbpfitness***

Made in the USA
Charleston, SC
25 April 2013